I0440711

Inside ADHD:

What It *Feels* Like and How to Use It Productively

Cedric David Benton Bluman

PRINTED IN CANADA

ISBN-13-978-1508807032

ISBN-10:1508807035

10-10-10 PUBLISHING

MARKHAM, ONTARIO

CANADA

CONTENTS

CONTENTS

FOREWORD

I am excited to endorse this book *INSIDE ADHD; WHAT IT FEELS LIKE AND HOW TO USE IT PRODUCTIVELY* by Cedric Bluman. It is both a unique personal description of his experience being labeled with this "diagnosis," as well as a thoughtful investigation into whether it is a "real" psychiatric diagnosis, a "high-tech" societal aberrancy or a different way of learning and living.

Cedric unapologetically explores his personal experiences and what it *feels* like to have a high-speed perception and being given the diagnosis of Attention Deficit Hyperactivity Disorder (ADHD). As a hyperactive child with language delay, he was diagnosed with Pervasive Developmental Delay, and later ADHD. In this brave and honest book: *Inside ADHD* he describes many different elements and symptoms of this alleged *disorder* in great detail. He also shares how ADHD manifested in his personal life growing up leading into adulthood, as well as *how* the psychological effects of the ADHD label and ADHD behavior affected him and his family.

He gives a raw account of his first-hand struggle being imprisoned and discouraged growing up with the label. He shares his experiences and how he transformed his life through embracing his inner negative self-judgements, and finding various disciplines strengthening his attention so that he discovered this high speed perceptivity was actually a beneficial trait for becoming creative and gifted at performance.   In turn, having learned to use his traits to his advantage, he seeks to encourage and guide you to recognize and understand the way of perceiving and living.

Cedric seeks to *empower* you to recognize those who have ADHD traits to help them find freedom from **vii** | P a g e being disorganized, distracted, discouraged, depressed, intimidated, and anxious.

He encourages you to back off from judging scatter-brained, inattentive behavior as negative and "hyperactive," and to query whether such traits are markers for a different way of perceiving, even a potential marker for heightened creativity.

This book will help you recognize, understand and appreciate such character traits in yourself or others:

- Do you have difficulty concentrating on what people say while they are speaking to you?
- Do you often leave your seat in situations where you are expected to remain?
- Do you have difficulty unwinding and relaxing when you have free time to yourself?
- Do you find yourself finishing sentences of people talking to you before they can?

- Do you put things off until the last minute?
- Do you depend on others to keep your life in order and attend to details for you?
- Do you have too many unfinished projects and dreams that your internal demons and even friends and family say are unrealistic?!

You live in the most technologically-savvy era of all time with more access to information online, via cell phone or television than ever imaginable…

Doctors are increasingly diagnosing children and adults with ADHD all across America and there is a marked rise in medical treatment.

Is excessive information helping or weakening our attention span? Or do you simply live in an impossibly distracting environment that steers your attention away at every moment?

So, what is ADHD? Is ADHD even a disorder?

Raymond Aaron
New York Times Bestselling Author

PREFACE

By Stephen Larsen, Ph.D. BCN, LMHC (NY State)
Psychology Professor Emeritus
State University of New York

Author and founder of the **Center for Symbolic Studies,** to carry on with the work of Joseph Campbell. Best known for his work in mythology, and being a pioneer in the field of neurofeedback, with particular focus on the Neurologically Sensitive Patient.

In this accessible and personal little book, Cedric Bluman has given us an offering not found elsewhere in the literature. Though there are a thousand books on ADD (ADHD), they are usually accounts by people wishing to inform parents and teachers about how to deal with the inattentive children they encounter in their daily parenting or teaching roles. But I know of very few accounts of what it *feels* like to be inside the skin of the ADD person.

I first met Cedric at about age 9, a very distractible little boy whose "motor" was apparently running far too fast. He scared and confused his parents and challenged his teachers. The LENS form of neurofeedback that I practiced then had a reputation for "speedy successes" with ADD. And Cedric *did* improve, but it was hard to get in the regular weekly treatments indicated, because the family lived seventy miles away, and both his parents were working professionals. Sometimes I thought it was hard to see any effect of our work together. But little Cedric had an "ace up his sleeve," that was destined not only to ameliorate his symptoms, but see him successfully through school, and ultimately college graduation. (Beyond enumerating difficult *symptoms*, such as anxiety, distractibility, sleep difficulties, etc., I seek to identify patients' strengths and gifts as grounds to build on for the future.)

Cedric had a passion for playing the piano.

The piano is good training for ADD in a variety of ways. Reading music requires a very particular kind of attention that many musicians never master. It involves both left and right hemispheres in an interactive dance. In addition to technical dexterity and proficiency there is also an emotional component of communicating the composer's intent. And, as I have observed over the years since I first met him, Cedric is full of passion for whatever he does.

When he had played a few simple classical pieces for me I knew he had an exquisite talent for music. He memorized well, and I knew that "keeping time" could help "slow down his motor." Fortunately, I have a grand piano in my therapy center meeting room, and I had him play for me almost every time I saw him. It was an ideal complement to our intermittent schedule of Neurofeedback treatments. I could hear how each note; and he loved their sounds, was itself a form of "feedback." In fact, I have come to believe, in part with Cedric's help, that music should probably be an integral part of any kind of brain training.

The book is first-hand and personal. It is based on real-life experience. Cedric does not hold back from how difficult at times his disability has been for him. But each time I have gone to a music recital or concert to hear him play, I have been rewarded. I can hear his progress in the music.

As with any form of therapy or self-improvement, there must be an emotional as well as mental and attentional component. Now he has added still another component to his communication repertoire: this book. I invite the reader to judge for him/herself whether Cedric's communication in this medium is as good as his primary arts (music and acting/filmmaking). I believe you will be rewarded.

Introduction

Writing this book helped me come to question my diagnosis that I received as a child of Attention Deficit Hyperactivity Disorder (ADHD). I am concerned that it became a crutch for me while growing up: an excuse for negligent behavior, as well as a belief that I could not perform optimally.

A diagnosis that hurts self-esteem and convinces you that you can't function without medication does not seem helpful to anyone. I think if a psychiatrist or a doctor, or anyone in an authoritative position, tells a patient they can't function well because of an attention disorder, it will probably trigger anxiety or hopelessness, enabling the patient to view themselves as a victim.

In fact, I wonder if ADD/ADHD should be classified as a mental disorder at all. Does it need to be "cured?" How can we be sure this is a problem originating in "attention deficiency" since the parents, therapists, and doctors are themselves subjective, trying to suppress, correct, or eradicate disruptive behavior?

I also wonder if ADHD is an over-diagnosed American phenomenon. In other cultures, psychotropic drugs are nowhere near as popular as in the US, and the diagnosis of ADHD is significantly less. Maybe it's more a matter of how parents and teachers in other countries discipline children at a young age.

I wish to share with anyone, what it *feels* like to have been labeled with ADD/ADHD. This book will hopefully help anyone with ADD/ADHD, and their loved ones to transform their approach to this alleged disorder and weigh a variety of options before considering buying prescriptions.

My aim in this book is to explore ADD/ADHD: to shed light on what it feels like to be diagnosed, and to prove that labeling certain behaviors and creativity as a problem is both counter-productive limiting creativity and self-expression. I believe there are ways to rewire negative thought processes in the mind with discipline and encouragement. Structure and a sense of meaning in a person's life helps develop creativity, instead of discouragement and depression.

What Is ADD/ADHD?

Attention Deficit Disorder (ADD) / Attention Deficit Hyperactivity Disorder (ADHD) is characterized by inattention and impulsiveness that is severe enough to impair academic, social, and occupational functioning. ADD children appear unfocused and unmotivated, while the hyperactive ones disrupt activities. While the causes are unknown, genetics and environmental factors are suspected influences.[1] In the *Diagnostic and Statistical Manual of Mental Disorders V* (DSM V), the classification of a child with ADD/ADHD

---

[1] Gaby, *Nutritional Medicine*, 1015.

requires that the symptoms be present by age twelve years.

PART 1   <u>ADHD from The Outside</u>

Parents, Teachers & Observers' Perspectives

Many young children by nature are uncontrollable, adventurous or impulsive—constantly on the go between activities. However, if they stand out as being particularly wild or difficult to teach in a classroom, they tend to be diagnosed with ADHD. Medication to "cure the problem" is usually suggested, since teachers and parents become frustrated. Teachers wish to control the child in the classroom, and parents want to cooperate with the education system (as well as control their own home environment).

The BBC documentary, *Living With ADHD* on YouTube, captured the lives of a few families with children diagnosed with ADHD, showing how these parents are faced with the apparently impossible task of controlling their kids.

Such hyperactivity has a huge impact on the parents, who usually feel their child won't listen to them, thus, injuring the esteem of both parents, as well as the child. The child also notices his/her parents' disappointment and bewilderment. A vicious cycle of behavioral and emotional chaos ensues.

When ADHD is diagnosed by "reliable" professionals, it usually results in a resounding shock of relief for the whole family. Parents are satisfied with an answer to their child's unique behavioral adjustments.[2]

Some physicians have seen ADHD as a diagnosis that pathologizes childhood behavior and makes symptoms seem more drastic than they might be. Physicians might see ADHD as a way of masking the detection of other, more important problems (aside from the behavioral symptoms); such as analyzing whether ADHD is a learning disorder.[3]

However, the diagnosis of ADHD may be inaccurate since symptoms of ADHD are also found in anxiety and depression. Also confounding, ADHD is often associated with many other comorbidities such as dyslexia and oppositional defiant disorder (the child is hostile, disobedient, and extremely difficult to discipline). Some psychologists believe children develop ADHD because they are constantly being reprimanded. Others believe exposure to environmental toxins, chemicals, food additives and dyes in foods trigger hypersensitivity and hyperactivity.

---

[2] Harrison-Hanley and Sussman, *Living With ADHD*.
[3] McLean Hospital, *Research Community: News*, January 8, 2003, cited in Null and Feldman, *Beyond Conventional Therapies*, 77.

Russell Barkley Ph.D., a professor of psychiatry specializing in ADHD, sees it as "Time Blindness" or "Temporal Neglect Syndrome." Barkley observed that the ADHD diagnosis is made when the child's behavior affects learning ability. He hypothesizes that kids/teenagers with ADHD live in the moment. He states that ADHD is a disorder of *performance*, not an attention deficit, but an *intention* deficit (inattention to details and future outcomes). They have trouble persisting and struggle with completing tasks because of their inability to perceive value in future or tangible results. This makes them susceptible to distraction, taking their attention away from what should be done at that time.[4] Thus, ADHD does not reflect an impairment in a person's competency or intelligence. It disrupts performance, goalsetting, and time management. Barkley is a very influential spokesperson for ADHD and is affiliated with the pharmaceutical industry. He is against biofeedback and is a heavy advocate for prescribing stimulant medication instead of biofeedback (Neurofeedback) which will be elaborated on later.

Many ADHD people experience pressure and constant angst to get things done. But for a multitude of reasons or excuses, they fail to follow through on tasks; distracted by persisting, internal negative voices that rattle inside the mind. This habit can begin in childhood, inhibiting

---

[4] Barkley, "Advances in Understanding."

productivity and causing them to feel "scatter brained."

Homework, career planning, and setting goals are usually impossible to complete because they feel lost. The future is too far off, perhaps something to fear, something to avoid thinking about. Video- gaming, television and leisure activities provide instant gratification for hours and help distract from those intimidating thoughts and goals for the future. This can actually be a form of *hyperfocusing*: "…the experience of deep and intense concentration in some people with ADHD. ADHD is not necessarily a deficit of attention, but rather a problem with regulating one's attention span to desired tasks. So, while mundane tasks may be difficult to focus on, others may be completely absorbing. An individual with ADHD who may not be able to complete homework assignments or work projects may instead be able to focus for hours on video games, sports, or reading."[5]

While it appears, the parents are the victims of their child's inexplicably erratic behavior, the child is also in a bind; containing within himself/herself a plethora of overly-active, persistent self-depreciating thoughts that rattle in the brain that persist into adolescence.

---

[5] Porter, "ADHD and Hyperfocus."

ADD/ADHD in Adults

What happens to kids with ADHD leading to adulthood? Can adults develop ADHD/ADD later? Don't they all struggle feeling, operating, and avoiding appearing different than other people? Aren't they forced into lower paying jobs because of being viewed as "retarded" "untalented', "odd" "off" "unconventional" "weird" or "losers"?

Like the childhood diagnosis, ADHD in adults is also associated with trouble paying attention, focusing, prioritizing, and managing time and money.[6]

A survey of 2,000 adults by the ADHD Awareness Coalition, led by CHADD: The National Resource on ADHD (Nationally recognized authority on ADHD), ADHD Coaches Organization (ACO), ADDitude Magazine and Attention Deficit Disorder Association (ADDA) found 60% lost their job due to ADHD, with more than 36% reported having four or more jobs in the past ten years, and 6.5% have ten or more jobs within the past ten years."[7]

Medical analyst Dr. Jon Hallberg emphasized that diagnosing ADHD in adults is difficult, since it can be made based on symptoms and what is observed. He predicted that 50% of kids with ADHD will become adults with ADHD. Naturally, in adulthood, challenges of increased

---

[6] Beck, "Mind Games."
[7] Pierce, LuAnn. "Is Adult ADHD a Disability?"

responsibility and competition will expose problems with time management, distractibility, and productivity. As a result, the diagnosed individuals may start to believe they are cognitively impaired, while the undiagnosed adults may seek professional evaluation and medical treatment more, thinking they have ADHD despite not being diagnosed as a child. "ADHD diagnoses are becoming more popular as ways to explain things that aren't going well. For example, it could have to do with the modern expectation of constant multitasking."[8]

Hallberg states that "anyone can pop an Adderall pill and be productive. However, not all general healthcare providers are trained to analyze whether these symptoms are from anxiety or depression, instead of ADHD. Ideally, the diagnosis should be made by a trained therapist's thorough, lengthy (one to three hour) comprehensive evaluation."

Rebecca Hersher from National Public Radio's article "Do You Zone Out? Procrastinate? Might Be Adult ADHD"[9] points out how the World Health Organization in collaboration with psychiatrists developed questions to determine whether an adult might have ADHD. Below are examples of such questions used by therapists to diagnose and treat ADD/ADHD:

---

[8] MPR News, "Diagnosing Adult ADHD."
[9] Hersher, "Might Be Adult ADHD."

- How often do you have difficulty concentrating on what people say to you, even when they are speaking to you directly?
- How often do you leave your seat in meetings and other situations in which you are expected to remain seated?
- How often do you have difficulty unwinding and relaxing when you have time to yourself?
- When in a conversation, how often do you find yourself finishing the sentences of the people you are talking to before they can finish them themselves?
- How often do you put things off until the last minute?
- How often do you depend on others to keep your life in order and attend to details?

Is ADD/ADHD Increasing in Both Children and Adults?

ADHD is more common than doctors may have previously believed, according to statistics from the Center for Disease Control and Prevention (CDC). The CDC report (November 2013) showed that up to 11% of children aged 4–17 were diagnosed with ADHD at some point in their lives, with 8.4% between ages 3–17 years, making up 5.2 million in the United States.

There have been 7.3 million ambulatory visits with ADD/ADHD as the primary diagnosis for families fretting over their children's behavior.

It is estimated that 1–3% of school age children have full-blown ADHD while 5–10% have partial ADHD.[10]

Some believe that 2/3 of children's symptoms persist into adulthood.[11,12] According to the National Resource on ADHD (CHADD), analysis of parent-reported data from the National Health Interview Survey (NHIS) 2011–2013 found 9.5% of children ages 4–17 years were diagnosed with ADHD: 2.7% of children ages 4–5, 9.5% of children ages 6–11, 11.8% of children ages 12–17. (Pastor. 2015)

Furthermore, the American Psychiatric Association emphasizes that the diagnosis of ADHD is not an easy one to make because the symptoms of ADHD are like those of many other childhood disorders. ADHD is often associated with other, comorbid conditions such as anxiety, communication disorders, brain trauma, depression, mood, conduct (oppositional defiant) and learning disorders—making ADHD more difficult to diagnose. (NIH; Tom Insel T M.D, 2014)

Analysis of prescription use also suggests there is an increase in ADD/ADHD diagnoses. According to the National Center for Health Statistics, 7.5% of U.S. children between ages 6–17 were taking medication for "emotional or behavioral difficulties" in 2011–2012. European

---

[10] Null and Feldman, "Beyond Conventional Therapies," 75.
[11] Robbins, "Paying Attention," 131.
[12] Barkley, "Advances in Understanding."

countries have also increased their use of methylphenidate drugs. According to the International Narcotics Control Board: Belgium, Germany, Iceland and the Netherlands increased use of methylphenidate drugs by 150–350% in a recent five-year period.[13]

According to Carolyn Gregoire's (2014) article *Worldwide ADHD Rates Are Higher Than Ever, And It Might Be America's Fault:* "…in the journal Social Science and Medicine, Conrad and colleague Meredith Bergey investigated the growth of ADHD diagnoses in five countries where ADHD diagnosis and treatment rates increased dramatically—the United Kingdom, Germany, France, Italy and Brazil. In Germany, for instance, prescription ADHD drugs increased from 10 million daily doses in 1998 to *53 million* in 2008. In the UK, stimulant-treatment for ADHD increased from under 200,000 prescriptions in 1991 to 1.58 million in 1995, according to data cited in the paper. These rates mirror the United States, where ADHD diagnoses have risen by almost 25% in a decade."[14]

PART 2   Problems with Diagnosing

Controversy: Is ADD/ADHD a Disorder?

A variety of assessment tools and rating scales are used to diagnose ADD/ADHD, including

---

[13] Null and Feldman, "Beyond Conventional Therapies," 75.
[14] Gregoire, "Worldwide ADHD Rates."

the Connors'/CADS scales and the numerous diagnostic criteria presented in the American Psychiatric Association's *Diagnostic and Statistical Manual of Mental Disorders*, Fifth Edition (DSM-5).

However, a big problem with such diagnostic assessments is that they are not definitive. A Consensus Statement was released in 1998 stating "there is no independent valid test for ADHD."[15] The National Institute of Health NIH indicates that the diagnosis of ADHD is more reliable through a methodical interview process with a patient.

Dr. William Carey, Clinical Professor of Pediatrics at the University of Pennsylvania School of Medicine, argues that ADHD is "...an oversimplified grouping of a complex and variable set of normal but incompatible temperamental variations; difficulties in learning, problems in school function and behavior, and sometimes neurological immaturity. A great variety of children's problems are being *compressed* into a single label: ADD/ADHD. Consequently, teachers, physicians and psychologists frequently do not agree and offer differing opinions about whether a specific child has the condition."

---

[15] "Diagnosis and Treatment of Attention Deficit Hyperactivity Disorder (ADHD): Consensus Statement," November 16, 1998, https://consensus.nih.gov/1998/1998attentiondeficithyperactivitydisorder110html.htm, cited in Null and Feldman, "Beyond Conventional Therapies," 76.

ADHD appears to affect five functions of the brain:

1) Inhibition and interference control
2) Nonverbal working memory (sensing of the self)
3) Verbal working memory (private self-speech)
4) Emotional and motivational self-regulation
5) Planning and problem solving[16]

Even more confusing, many other psychological diagnoses share the same symptoms: autism, anxiety, depression, and more. Kids with ADHD don't necessarily come from hectic environments or traumatic familial situations. Doctors and scientists are still unsure of how these symptoms arise in children. Bruce Levine M.D. is concerned that more and more people whose behavior is well within a range of normal are being "pathologized."[17]

Classification of ADHD Types: "Common Inattentive," "Hyperactive," "Combined" and Pervasive Developmental Delay

Since 1994, different types of "attention" disorders have been recognized:

---

[16] Barkley, "*Behavioral Inhibition.*"
[17] Levine, "Why the Rise?"

- Pervasive Common: inattentive with minimal hyperactivity and impulsive behavior—ADD

- Hyperactive: compulsive with hyperactivity—ADHD

- Combined: ADD/ADHD with both features

- Development Delay

Studies indicate 30–50% of children with ADHD are only "inattentive." Barkley hypothesizes that such "inattentive-types represent a separate disorder from ADHD."

<u>Common Type</u>

The "common" inattentive ADD child can be described as: daydreaming, spacey, slow-moving, lethargic, sluggish motor/cognitive, easily confused, error prone when information processing, poorly focused with selective attention, socially withdrawn, not impulsive, and having a small selection of friends. They lack the 'hyperkinetic' behavioral patterns, and instead frequently fantasize and daydream. They have trouble engaging in tasks and organizing. They rarely show aggression or oppositional defiant disorder and conduct disorder, making the diagnosis difficult to detect.

These "common" type ADD children struggle on an emotional level because they tend to live a repressed, unexpressed existence during their childhood and adolescence because of how undetectable the symptoms are to others. They are at greater risk for anxiety or depression, impaired academic performance, drug use, and conduct problems. According to Barkley, the "inattentive" type children and adults benefit the most from stimulants and perhaps because these medications temporarily relieve anxiety and depression symptoms.[18]

Hyperactive Type

Characteristics of ADHD children include hyperactivity, restlessness, irritability, curiosity, constantly being in motion doing many things without satisfaction. Young children who are particularly adventurous or impulsive may be erroneously diagnosed with ADHD.

Combined Type

The combined ADD/ADHD diagnoses appears at a young age. As these children transition to adulthood they have higher rates of antisocial personality disorders, depression, substance abuse, and adult psychopathy (lacking empathy, conscience, guilt, remorse).

---

[18] Barkley, "Advances in Understanding."

Pervasive Development Disorder

Pervasive Developmental Disorder (PDD) is a subcategory of ADD/ADHD where the child fails to meet developmental milestones from an early age. The child does not maintain eye contact with others, is unable to creep or crawl as a baby, and learns to walk and speak later than children his own age). In 2011, scientists abandoned this classifying approach, claiming symptoms and behaviors vary widely in the ADHD spectrum and should be individualized for each patient. Brain-scanning techniques to diagnose ADHD were deemed 'premature and impractical' due to expenses and lack of guidelines interpreting the brain scans.[19]

PART 3   Exploring Causes

What is Attention?

"In the early 20th Century, William James pointed out that *attention* was the pivotal mechanism not only of consciousness, but of learning, character development, and creative life fulfillment."[20] When people do what they "love," attention is easily mobilized, and daily practices and dedications are honed and sought out.

---

[19] Larsen, *The Neurofeedback Solution*, 144.
[20] Larsen, *The Neurofeedback Solution*, 145.

A great mystery of hyperactivity lies in the ADHD child/adult's ability to *hyperfocus* in one area of field of study and be completely undistracted or uninterested in another, for hours at a time. This might be a gift useful in developing a talent or creative projects, or a curse predisposing to addictive behavior and feeling very dissatisfied in many work environments.

Excessive videogames and screen time; internet sites, television shows, excessive phone use, movies—can be very *distracting* activities that can negatively affect anyone's capacity to pay attention. Excessive stimulation with these modalities can numb and entrap the attention within the confines of a screen and provide instant gratification, provoke isolation and escapism, assisting detachment and lapses of attention—and this does not just pertain to the diagnosed ADD/ADHD person.

Just because a person struggles with attention doesn't mean they don't have ambition or a thirst for knowledge. Maybe it's really because they just may not have yet found what genuinely rivets their attention. If they possess a desire for knowledge or training, their curiosity will wonderfully never be quenched because of their endless thinking patterns!

Projects or careers that involve their passions, things that fascinate the individual, will unquestionably motivate the "inattentive" person to follow through and complete the process with care. And hopefully, like music did for me, intense tutelage and discipline from passionate teachers and mentors can help develop attention and concentration.

Is ADD/ADHD Rooted in Anxiety and Fear?

If fear triggers anxiety, could fear and anxiety stimulate the ADD/ADHD person to the point that they can't function? Or could fear *potentially* become a catalyst for an increase in energy for performance? For example, meeting deadlines and goals?

Many people with ADD/ADHD do not possess *enough* anxiety to become stressed; which could explain their passive behavior regarding responsibilities or obstacles. Or there can be the opposite condition; an incapacity to strive to perform at a high level because of anxiety and fear.

In Dale Carnegie's *How to Win Friends and Influence People,* he quotes Charles Schwab: "there is nothing else that so kills the ambitions of a person as criticism from superiors. I never criticize anyone, I believe in giving a person incentive to work.[21] Carnegie also claims that people will aspire to great things, potentially go insane and become outrageously depressed, all based on fear of being insignificant.

ADHD individuals are often criticized and ridiculed throughout childhood into adulthood for many different reasons: lateness on submitting

---

[21] Carnegie, *How to Win Friends and Influence People*, TK.

assignments, irresponsible behavior, lack of attention, etc.—which can take major toll on their self-esteem.   I believe that the desire to feel important is an inherent human need that becomes apparently unattainable for anyone who has been told their whole life "you *can't* stay on task, pay attention, or complete projects. You will never be successful being the way you are." Emotions of panic and plummeting self-esteem can also arise as a result of competing against other people who the discouraged person deems as "superior," based on financial success, fame, popularity, and creativity, whatever.

Thus, traumatic memories of people from one's past telling you, "you're stupid and incompetent" can majorly affect attention and performance in the moment.

I also firmly believe that self-treatment with stimulant medication (and abuse) can lead to a false feeling of importance, as well as physical and psychological dependence. Perhaps this is the main reason self-medication with stimulants occurs: so that the person can *feel* like they have attention or feel less distracted. On stimulant medication, they might feel less fearful, less doubtful, and more confident in their abilities.

Unfortunately, in my opinion, trying to feel important or focused under the influence of a stimulant is not reality. It is not genuine success. The euphoric, stimulating effects of psychotropic drugs makes one *feel* successful, but doesn't necessarily make a person successful regarding the quality of work, or productivity while on the medication.

Anxiety provokes tunnel vision; fight or flight emotional responses, akin to claustrophobia with uncomfortable sensations. It can feel like the environment is closing in. Powerful, ruthlessly cruel introspection and self-deception can take place. Your heart palpitates, and you second guess your every word and action. I believe such negative thought patterns are learned. How many people with ADD/ADHD end-up seeing themselves as victims being attacked?

Thus, a defensive, fight or flight reaction can be aroused whenever they perceive they are in the presence of a superior colleague/teacher, or anyone they perceive as criticizing or ridiculing. It becomes hard to foster and make new relationships when the learned response is self-defense and fight-or-flight. As a result of assuming that people see the worst or are about to lecture them, the ADD/ADHD person relearns this internal response again and again, accepts it, and submits repetitively inside into a self-contained, tormented version of themselves.

Anxiety is associated with many other disorders: Depression, Obsessive Compulsive Disorder (OCD), Post-Traumatic Stress Disorder (PTSD), and so on. The 'generalized anxiety disorder' is when anxiety attends every aspect of a person's life daily in response to specific or general situations; from public speaking, to sports, performing musically, socializing, etc.[22]

These anxieties tend to eradicate liberation, self-acceptance, and awareness. These neurological (physiological and psychological) phobias control a person's brain and sense of empowerment (what one believes they can or cannot do), thus denying an individual to express themselves.

Anxiety induces intense panic within. The physiological symptoms of anxiety include butterflies in stomach, heart pounding, and weakness of breath, dry mouth, clammy skin, and the feeling of death.[23] These sensations manipulate the body and make a person feel like giving up or shying away from many activities or opportunities in their life, creating many inhibitions and preconceived notions.

Furthermore, if we deduce that fear is a major component of triggering anxiety and other ADD/ADHD symptoms, we can use that to help the child/adult. In conversing with ADD/ADHD people struggling personally and financially, it might be more helpful to analyze their dysfunctional lifestyle by asking: "What is bothering you? What are you afraid of? How can you face this fear and find a solution? Can I talk to you for a minute?" instead of carelessly ordering them to do things, dismissing them, and verbally mocking or abusing them.

---

[22] Larsen, *The Neurofeedback Solution*, 168.
[23] Larsen, *The Neurofeedback Solution*, 168.

For me personally, heading into college and even post-graduation, I realize now that I had many flashbacks of interactions with people throughout my life. These moments in time were subtle; they maybe even felt insignificant when they happened. But these impressions and memories certainly had a role in my development: I can recall many instances of cracking jokes, people laughing, people rolling their eyes, turning away, pointing fingers and lecturing/talking down to me—small human gestures and body movements that can easily go unnoticed, such as smirks, mocking comments. But over time, those images haunted me. I was afraid and angered at the idea of being laughed at, having someone point their finger at me, turning their back away, walking away, calling me "stupid."

I do believe that our memories and negative altercations with people—yes, everyone is different and there are many different circumstances and forms of abuse or discord—can heavily impact our view of strangers and associates/friends. Carrying these memories can certainly provoke anger and anxiety and can force us into feeling uneasy, on-guard, vengeful, isolated…all contributing to the impulse to hide and protect ourselves from meeting new people, making amends, and learning new things.

Traumatic Brain Injury, Head Trauma and ADHD

Traumatic Brain Injury (TBI) also causes difficulties with organization, time management, sleep, mood instability, conflicting energy patterns, and trouble planning or working towards a goal, bodily pain, headaches, and chronic fatigue.[24] Maureen Salamon notes that "the effects of the TBI may be additive to those of ADHD. TBI results in more than 7,000 deaths, 60,000 hospitalizations and 600,000 emergency room visits annually in the United States."[25] According to the Brain Injury Resource Center in the United States there are an estimated 300,000 sports related TBI's per year."[26]

ADHD and TBI seem viciously linked. Dr. Stephanie Greene, an assistant professor of neurological surgery at Children's Hospital of Pittsburgh, says "Part of the problem with children with ADHD is that they often have poor impulse control, which means that they are at higher risk of sustaining a TBI by engaging in risk-taking behaviors in daily life, separate from sports. When risky sports are added to the already elevated risk of traumatic brain injury, the chances of a child sustaining a traumatic brain injury becomes unacceptably high."[27]

Dr. Larsen suggests that the idea of heroism—such as jousting and fights to the death

---

[24] Ibid., 198.
[25] Salamon, *"Longer-Lasting Head Injury."*
[26] Larsen, *The Neurofeedback Solution*, 224.
[27] Salamon, *"Longer-Lasting Head Injury."*

(as depicted in films, videogames, sports and entertainment, and more)—has contributed to why children today are prone to physical accidents. In addition, our culture is fascinated with sports spectatorship and adoration of athletes.[28]

Discordant Home Life & ADD/ADHD

As a child, I witnessed verbal abuse and arguing between my parents, who eventually divorced. There were also other familial issues going on; my grandparents became progressively ill, and there was a major divide in our extended family that lasted many years, emotionally and financially impacting all of us.

My parents were not home a lot and my brother, and I were cared for by babysitters. While I grew up in Westchester and had a pleasant, nurturing upbringing by most standards, in looking back on my childhood, I cannot deny how difficult parental disagreements, parental absence, and a chaotic household were for me. As a result, I now realize how understandably scattered I was.

Parental disagreements, loud fights or verbal attacks aimed at each other or the child, can reinforce distractible, anxious behavior. It can force the child to rebel or impulsively try to escape these memories through other means, especially in adolescence and adulthood. I strongly believe that a difficult home life can be a reason why children

---

[28] Larsen, *The Neurofeedback Solution*, 222.

engage in reckless behavior and seek out psychotropic or other drugs (Marijuana, LSD, Cocaine, and more) to *suppress* or blot out traumatic or depressing memories and emotions.

PART 4   Treatment

Controversies in Managing ADHD

How to *treat* ADHD is a controversial subject. Many doctors and therapists advocate stimulant medications. Those who encourage drug treatment have not been well-received by many therapists and practitioners in the ADHD field. Below are some valuable arguments presented by Teresa Gallagher from *Born to Explore; The Other Side of ADHD, Refuting Against the Severities and Hubbub of ADHD*. They are concerned that the early childhood developmental stages may be adversely affected by medications. Overprescribed drugs, neglect, and verbal or physical abuse all can wreak harmful, potentially permanent effects. The child cannot decipher what is right and wrong because of persisting, cognitive confusion.

Richard Bromfield, Ph.D., a psychologist at Harvard Medical School says, "Studies show that Ritalin prescribing fluctuates dramatically depending on how parents and teachers perceive 'misbehavior' and how tolerant they are of it. I know of children who have been given Ritalin more to subdue them than to meet their needs—a practice that recalls the opium syrups used to soothe noisy infants in London a century ago."

National Association of School Psychologists (NASP), with 13,000 accredited members, states in their NASP Communique, Volume 29, and Number 1: "We believe that the construct of ADD/ADHD has come to act like a set of blinders. Once an educator observes that a child has a perceived degree of difficulty attending, he/she tends to ask whether the child has an 'Attention Deficit Disorder.' The many other potential sources of inattention are often bypassed and not even considered. For example, has the child experienced any trauma and/or is she/he anxious or depressed? Could the child's temperament and/or personality style be the source of inattention? Do the child's nutritional habits support a well settled and attentive approach to learning? Are there any medical conditions that make it difficult for the child to focus and settle down? Are there ecological or contextual factors that may be implicated in attentional problems? Is the child's learning/interactional environment disordered?"

Peter R. Breggin, M.D., author of *Talking Back to Ritalin* said: "In my practice of psychiatry, I am frequently consulted about children who are taking three, four, and sometimes five psychiatric drugs, including medications that are FDA-approved only for the treatment of psychotic adults. The drug treatment typically began when the children developed conflicts with adults at home or at school. In retrospect, the conflicts could easily have been resolved by interventions such as family counseling or individualized educational approaches. Usually under pressure from a school, the parents instead acquiesced to put their child on stimulants prescribed by psychiatrists, family physicians, or pediatricians."

Treating ADD/ADHD with Medication

Pharmaceutical drugs may provide the user with artificial/temporary confidence, but when the drug's effects wear off, so does the confidence. Some users might believe over time with extended use that they cannot live or function *without* the drugs. Thus, they may secretly feel incapable, worthless, and stupid. While stimulant medications certainly can help performance (such as Adderall, Ritalin, Vyvanse or any form of amphetamines), these drugs can be addictive and have adverse side effects.

It seems likely that ADD/ADHD is over-diagnosed and probably overmedicated. In fact, analysis of prescription use is another way to estimate the increase in ADD/ADHD diagnoses. According to the National Center for Health Statistics, 7.5% of U.S. children between ages 6–17 were taking medication for "emotional or behavioral difficulties" in 2011–2012.

Children are typically prescribed a low dosage and the dosage increases as they get older, perpetuating the psychological and physical need for the medication. According to American

Addiction Centers, 50 million prescription stimulant drugs like Adderall were dispensed in 2011 to treat symptoms of attention deficit hyperactivity disorder, or ADHD. This represents an almost 40% rise in these prescriptions since 2007, according to the Drug Enforcement Agency (DEA).

Many psychologists and clinicians are prescribing stimulant medications. According to the U.S. Centers for Disease Control and Prevention, as of 2011—11% of people ages 4–17 diagnosed with ADHD, had access to stimulant medications. (NIH, The Science of Drug Abuse and Addiction, 2014)

Sales of these prescription drugs (e.g., Strattera and Concerta to Ritalin, Vyvanse, and Adderall) have been soaring, treating children, teenagers, and adults.[29] These drugs contain methylphenidate, amphetamine, and dextroamphetamine, which affect dopamine transport into the brain.

Stimulant drugs speed up thought. Processing becomes less effortful. Tasks that were formerly perceived as impossible, overly challenging, or distasteful seem more pleasurable and doable (Larsen, Stephen, 2012, pg. 151). Meanwhile, these drugs have become increasingly popular with all ages in the last twenty years.

In the documentary, *The Untold Story of Psychotropic Drugging: Making a Killing,* Gwen Olson (former drug sales representative) states,

---

[29] Barkley, "Advances in Understanding."

"there is an unholy alliance between psychiatry and pharmaceutical sales..." Dr. Gary Gordon states, "The psychiatrists today admit they can't cure these mental illnesses and are therefore going to 'manage' your illness by using a drug."[30] Throughout the documentary, various psychologists and clinicians interviewed describe the twisted methods of the pharmaceutical industry and their massive impact on American lives....

PART 5   ADD/ADHD from The INSIDE

People with ADD/ADHD can experience an exhausting array of thought processes throughout the day; scrambled, internalized voices that usually spark negativity or feeling scattered. These thought processes can be intensified by intruding reminders about what hasn't been accomplished or scheduled, what hasn't been fixed, where or how to progress professionally, and who to consult. Time is always getting away—there is so much to do and seemingly never enough time. This can be both a recipe for increased productivity and also Basically, time management can seem absurd.

Here's an example based on personal experience:

---

[30] Burwell and Stith, *Untold Story.*

"Okay, it's 7:30am and it's important that I go jogging today because cardio will lead to weight loss, is a way to release endorphins, get rid of toxins, and can help me function and fall asleep at a reasonable hour later tonight. But I know I have to be at the office for check-in by 9. So, I should make eggs and coffee, go for a run. No wait, I should run first but I'm supposed to have this assignment completed before I get in the office. Why didn't I do that last night? Okay, complete the chart lists for my boss now and show them to him by afternoon! Maybe I can fit the jog in later in the day because its already been twenty minutes and I'm losing time boiling the water for the eggs and I can't find my pants and the appropriate dress shirt to go with—and god dammit, where did I put my socks? I need to file papers and go to the bank later and deposit that check, can't forget—okay I guess there's time for a set of pushups! But I probably shouldn't do two things at once—oh my God, I forgot to email Sharron! Do that right now and then eat the eggs—did I take them out of the refrigerator or are they overcooked? I guess I won't eat breakfast, then. But without a balanced breakfast I won't have high energy. Wow, there goes my morning workout, I'm never gonna lose weight...oh crap, my shirt is at the dry cleaners...this is why you're not getting promoted because you can't even put on clothes properly, you idiot!"

Inside, ADD/ADHD can feel like mental/emotional "high-alert" prison. Being labeled as cognitively impaired is discouraging. Teachers, bosses, family and friends who jokingly comment or intend to insult an ADD ADHD person for being scatter-brain, further reinforces the conviction of being worthless and different than "normal" people. It can also lead to other psychological detriments for that individual; they may become antisocial, depressed, vengeful and frustrated towards people—all from the feelings and memories associated with being insulted by others. Thus, these labelings can lead a person into living a reclusive, angry, and lonely existence.

What It's Like to Have ADHD: My Story

While I was in my mother's womb, she was hyper-productive, developed premature labor around 28 weeks and was treated with Terbutaline—which is like caffeine—which made her even more hyperactive and speedy than she already was, despite being forced to bed rest. I was born slightly prematurely, developed an infection, and was put into the ICU in a neonatal incubator for the first 2 weeks of my life, getting intravenous antibiotics and blood tests every day.

My mom says that when I was maybe four or five years old, while driving in our car at night I saw lights on the nearby bridge and blurted, "Oh Mom, the acupuncture needles they used were horrible!" She realized that the lights must have triggered a memory of being in the Neonatal ICU with the night lights there, because I had never been treated with acupuncture.

I was with my mom every day until she had to go back to work when I was seven months old. On that day, I skipped crawling and all of a sudden,

I stood up and cruised around on my feet. I later had speech delay.

Then at age three, I suddenly recited every word of the Robert Louis Stevenson poem "When I Go to Bed at Night" from start to finish. My uncle Jean Cieslak, a specialist in teaching handicapped children, noticed that I did not make eye contact and urged my parents to seek therapy immediately. I was then diagnosed with Pervasive Developmental Delay (PDD). I also did not use my thumbs to grasp. My parents sought help from numerous practitioners; psychologists, physical and occupational therapists. We even tried Primal Scream therapy (which I don't recall).

I have been told that my childhood behavior was considered abnormal or 'off-the-wall.' I recall being analyzed by physicians, psychotherapists, neurologists, and more. Although I did not understand what was happening, I did perceive that there was something unusual over the years that my parents and I had innumerable family conferences, detentions, and meetings during class and after school. I was very sociable in pre-school class settings but spent a lot of time by myself once school was over.

In addition, throughout my childhood, I hit my head many times: on pavement, rocks, and collisions with friends in little league sports. I even fell head-first out of a shopping cart onto concrete around age two or three. I recall being constantly in movement; drawn to fast-moving, thrill-triggering activities, jumping off roofs, rolling down hills and colliding into tree branches and rocks, zooming away on sleds in winter, flailing in leaves in the fall—activities that many children do. TBI accidents might explain a lot of my struggles.

Various physicians and developmental specialists identified that I had "processing deficits" (i.e. that I did not quickly "catch" or understand concepts quickly). I had a different way of learning; I was considered a "right-brained" person.

As a child, I was scolded (understandably) by my teachers for bad class behavior and negligence with homework and time management. I wanted to improve. But based on years of punishment and verbal criticism, I learned to fear punishment, fearing even the mere thought of being punished or put-down by anyone in authority (parents, peers, schoolteachers).

I went to many counselors and therapists for my lack of attention and bad behavior in middle-school and high school. I continued to go to psychotherapists, faculty evaluations, checklists, detention. I was unable to stay in a chair through a whole class until the end of 5th grade. Struggling with staying attentive in a classroom without being distracted continued throughout middle school and high school.

I was officially diagnosed with ADHD during middle school and was allowed more time taking exams. As a teen, I became self-sabotaging and locked-up in my perception of my imperfections. This habitual process of self-loathing, like any behavioral pattern, became deeply ingrained and was very difficult to live with.

My Relationship with Time

Time always seemed (and still does) like something that is always "getting away." In adolescence and early adulthood, I experienced hyperbolic self-criticism and demonic thoughts: "I didn't accomplish anything today!!!" or "I didn't accomplish enough!!!" or "I never accomplish anything at all!!!" and "I'm a worthless piece of shit because I have so many deadlines and half-assed completed projects that could have been successful if I hadn't...blah blah blah!!!"

With all these racing thoughts, I always felt as if I was at a standstill. I felt discouraged by my lack of time management skills. Threats and discouraging remarks from my parents, teachers, and bosses, who repeatedly pointed out my failure to follow rules or instructions convinced me that I lacked motivation, discipline, and was unable to problem solve and plan.

I felt stupid, angry, and lost in high school. I would act out in class, try to entertain others by fooling and joking around, and didn't want to think about school assignments. As a result of constant joking around and unintentionally creating a bad reputation for myself, I was the "class clown."

Being brought up in a small private school environment and challenging negative issues at home (parents separating, grand-parents declining and dying, financial struggles and other things) may explain my holding onto relationships, many of which were superficial or were unhealthy.

Based on my adolescent experiences, I created an image or a façade of being an entertainer in my small school environment. I had an insatiable desire to seek approval from friends and peers; desperate for any form of attention, even if it meant making a fool of myself. As a result, some enjoyed my antics and befriended me as a source of pleasure or hilarity, and others simply judged and rejected me.

I was very wild in classes from middle school to the end of high school. Laughter, distraction, joking around with friends—was a form of escapism. Long-term goals—such as where I wanted to go to college or what I wanted to do as a career—were subjects I avoided thinking about. This was all due to deep feelings of insecurity, believing I couldn't pay attention and couldn't function at a high level academically, etc.

However, one positive influence occurred in my high-school senior year at Rockland Country Day School (RCDS). Seniors were required to work individually all year on a "Senior Project" they chose to create. I worked on writing a screen-play and directing, filming, and acting in a film. I loved working on it. I discovered that, regardless of the outcome or quality of the film, I was able to finish *something* from start to finish. It was a step in a positive direction.

During my freshman year I college, I continued to struggle with guilt and low self-esteem. I recognized that I had underachieved in high school. Negative thought processes left me feeling dejected and made making new friends very difficult. I missed opportunities to integrate myself into campus life. I found myself alone, on my own.

That's when I discovered my passion for classical music. It was at this time that I fell in love with piano. I'd been playing piano since age nine and had taken lessons, but it never meant anything to me and I didn't practice much at all. Now that I was on my own in college, it helped me to unwind and de-stress after classes and was an amazing outlet for self-expression.

I also started getting into abusive relationships. Some were self-pity relationships where I fought for the person's approval of me. They were relationships that revolved around: "please give me another chance! I know I made mistakes, I'm wretched, please forgive me, please help me; I want to be involved, to be liked and praised; please approve of me, I need your help and expertise…"

In fact, feeling victimized and pitying oneself usually leads to these abusive type relationships. People who feel guilty or lame about themselves tend to gravitate to people with inflated egos or who have garnered a respectable reputation. Or they tend to gravitate to low-self-esteem people just like them. These relationships are toxic, because no one should be worshipped, no one should have control over anyone. That isn't friendship or collaboration.   Since I was yearning for a disciplinary lifestyle, I confided and empowered friends who I perceived as "superior" role models to discipline and help guide me, thus, offering them an unhealthy power trip. I kept seeking people who would help "fix" and "improve" me. It was like I was searching for a guru, someone with all the answers. Unwittingly, I became attracted to relationships that reinforced and further cultivated my internal criticism and low self-esteem.

Then I heard about stimulant medications for focusing. College kids were always talking about it, describing it as a gateway drug, something that makes you more outgoing and focused on schoolwork. Frustrated at my own inability to maintain focus for an extended period, I asked to be treated with stimulant medications by my local doctor. Once I was introduced to Adderall, the powerful effects were hard to ignore.

My Bad Relationship with Adderall

My relationship with Adderall started when I was a sophomore in college. Growing up, I had a very sheltered upbringing. In college, I was introduced to Greek Life and bar hopping. I met many people from different walks of life. I was quickly knocked out of my little shell and introduced to completely new social strata.

These college kids spoke so differently than kids I had grown up with in Westchester and Rockland County. They had different musical and aesthetic tastes. These college frat boys nonchalantly knew the words to literally every rap or hip-hop song that came on during a party. I didn't know any trendy music and had a hard time "fitting in." I liked Classical Music and seldom listened to Drake, J. Cole, ASAP Rocky, or The Weeknd, to name a few artists. Nevertheless, I wanted social acceptance and attended to a lot of college parties in my Freshman year.

I also started to smoke pot. I found myself mixing on and off with groups of kids who I never thought existed outside the characters of *Easy Rider* and *Fear and Loathing in Las Vegas*. They were hippies, free spirits. The one thing that held all their relationships together was their love of drugs and mutual feelings of "highs and lows", addiction, and self-destruction.

In the beginning, I thought this process was fascinating. I wanted to observe and partake to feel accepted, like I was getting a "worldly" education. I never truly believed I was "one of a crowd." I also started talking like them, mingling with them, and doing what they were doing, to be socially accepted. Before I knew it (and I was in denial for some time), I was a pothead with even lower self-esteem without any ambition.

Adderall allegedly helped amplify performance and could make you do anything you want at a very high level. I watched some people at parties take the drug. They would confidently wash down drink after drink, scream or sing at the top of their lungs, start rap battles, talk a mile a minute. This state of elation was exciting; how could a pill induce such a state of euphoria?

Anyone who took it seemed extremely driven, borderline sociopathic—it seemed that nothing negative entered their personal bubble or could bruise their ego. I had to admit, I was curious about how ingesting a pill could simply make all attention deficits and life obstacles *fade away!*

One of the kids in my hall, who was prescribed Vyvanse, warned me about the drug. He'd been notably abusing his prescription for his ADHD. He blamed his lack of organization and academic competence on the disorder and his incapacity to pay attention. While I also was prescribed medication as a teen, my parents, skeptical and wary of the lack of research on long-term Adderall or amphetamine usage, were against prescription treatments. Thus, I never took any medication in my youth.

One day, I saw this same guy stooped over outside his dorm, nodding out like a heroin junky. He had a morbid, worn out expression smeared across his face. In that moment, that 18-year-old looked 70 years old. He shook his head exhausted and with a demonic smile, he explained how strung out he was feeling. He said, almost in a boasting tone, that he'd been awake for two days. He explained how he'd been writing songs, had missed all homework assignments and had skipped every single class that whole week. He said he knew he was going to flunk out this semester.

I told him, "Dude…just stop taking it, then." He assured me he would stop after he renewed his next prescription. Then he demonically laughed and said he had consumed a month's prescription in under two weeks. I couldn't understand how a person could inflict such self-harm. Well, not yet.

A few months later, I transferred to another college to study film. I still had a lethargic attitude, was apprehensive, and continued to struggle with organization and time management. I was smoking pot too much, which made me passive. I avoided writing or gathering people together to make ideas and films come to life because of the fear of failure and fear of rejection.

I realized that you are who you associated with. I hung out, yet again, in my new environment, with potheads. I was dependent on the "weed-state of mind." The fogginess had become normal. I self-medicated, instead of returning to psychotherapy or Neurofeedback (the treatment I had undergone frequently as a child to help normalize my brain waves). Distraction from my college responsibilities had become a mode of existence.

All of this was happening below the surface. I still believed I was people watching and gaining perspective. Thus, on this journey of self-discovery or quite frankly, chronic stupidity, I finally tried Adderall myself. The guy who introduced me to Adderall is now dead. He died from drug overdose.

I bought the pills through a dealer he knew. I ingested one pill...ten minutes later, I felt euphoric, sensational, and genuinely hopeful about my future life prospects. My anxiety quieted down. An inner instinct and sense of well-being permeated through my body. I thought in that moment: "Anything is possible in this beautiful world." I realized why they called this a "miracle drug."

I worked out in the gym that night for three hours straight and then I wrote five pages of a paper due for the next day. I wrote poems and planned some film concepts. I slept uncomfortably for a few hours. That month, I took Adderall a couple times. Every time the experience was immensely entertaining and rejuvenating.

However, now I think Adderall is like junk food for the soul.

I had become very focused on the piano and filmmaking. The drug taught me that inspiration is a force to be reckoned and that hard work presents the creator with a product; written material to work with and is conducive as opposed to having ideas contained and unpresented in one's head, where it doesn't actually exist. This is a major problem with ADHD people; they just tend to fail to write everything down that pops into their heads. As a result, they feel they are incompetent left with, or have nothing.

Adderall gave me a physical sense of elation, sensory pleasure and feelings of an inner tingling sensation; an artificial, enhanced feeling of joy or bliss. I felt like I had a divine purpose and reason to be alive in the world and the universe; like I was larger than life. The euphoric state of inspiration made me feel as if connected to a higher power. It's as if the drug-enthused performer puts on a show for God.

Short-acting Adderall lasts a couple of hours. Long-lasting Adderall is subtler; it's less emotional and physically riveting and lasts 8 to 10 hours. Either way, placebo effect or feeling high, I found homework, and menial tasks—writing a list, laundry, cleaning the dorm, showering and putting on clothes, walking to class—to be interesting and motivational. I felt more conscious and aware of what I was doing as opposed to feeling in a fog. Practicing piano and filmmaking were also less strenuous or boring and became exciting.

However, I began to notice when I "came down", and the drug effects began to wear off. I felt worse after taking a pill than when I began. I felt physically drained, irritable, hungry, and lonely.

On Adderall, my social anxiety was suppressed by frantic behavior. I spoke quickly and efficiently with people and assumed that my tone of voice and agitated personality were likeable, endearing, and exciting to others. I felt like a performer and an advisor; full of wit, intelligent thoughts, and great vibes that I wished to bestow upon people I came in contact with on campus. In limited doses. On my terms.

I found myself in a hurry to get to campus, get to class, get to work, and be productive. I always felt guilty that I wasn't utilizing my Adderall time wisely. I would avoid conversing or relating to others for too long to be productive while the effects of the drug were still intact. I felt that it would be a waste of money to pay for college and to be social. "That is something I could do anytime," I thought.

Months passed. I found myself slipping away from my friends. I noticed that people I interacted with could tell when I was having a great day, usually under the influence of stimulants, versus when I was in recovery from an all-nighter and not on stimulants. Eventually, I tried to avoid being seen in public sober.

Overtime, I began to abuse the doses and buy from various dealers more frequently. I found myself traveling outside my circle and calling multiple contacts off-campus many times a week to make sure I had a hookup. The money I earned at my retail job went towards my fix. I never went out partying or into NYC on weekends because of physical exhaustion, fear of never being productive enough. I was estranging myself from my friends and associates.

During these all-nighters, I would force myself to practice piano, study or workout— anything to keep from being quiet and still; keeping myself busy avoiding actual reflection about my life. I would lose three pounds in one day and gain it back in two days. Sometimes, I was unable to leave my bedroom from dehydration, depression, and exhaustion. I missed classes and submissions.

I kept going back to Adderall because the spurt of joy and willingness to be productive only seemed to arise when I was high. I was living a double life. There were nights when I would stare into a mirror, throw a pill down the toilet, and then moan in agony as I realized I'd thrown away a piece of my salvation. The second I'd decided to quit, a demonic voice inside would say insidiously, "*Chill man, just one more time, it's not a big deal…you need it.*" Then I would call a dealer immediately.

I remember outings with friends seemed forced and unnatural. I would find myself in a state of delirium and insomnia. Sometimes, when I was high, I would talk intimately about life with acquaintances I barely knew just because they asked me how my day was going. Many would nod hurriedly at me when we passed each other on campus because the connection or moment from the day before was false. I stopped working out with my gym buddies because I no longer had enough energy to lift weights or do cardio.

This lifestyle persisted during college semesters when Adderall was readily available, until breaks in the semester, when I came home.

This went on from sophomore year to senior graduation.

I would wait anxiously for the next opportunity for a dealer to contact me. Whatever it took; if the dealers were done with class, off work, finished with vacation—I was willing to meet them anywhere. I would drive hours to meet them. Adderall had become my only real source of pleasure in my life and without it, I couldn't conceive of a better life. The only sense of accomplishment I ever felt was when I was high.

I started overdosing and had a poor attitude about completing tasks and working sober. My Adderall addiction was at an all-time high. The scariest issue I had to deal with was my family and friends. While I'm sure they noticed my lack of intimacy and distant behavior, they couldn't detect *exactly* what was wrong. They probably thought it was simply youthful hormonal changes or my ADHD, anxious disposition. I embarked on a self-imposed, difficult senior semester. I decided to make a film about piano, give a piano recital, make a piano recording, write my senior thesis, and graduate from college.

I believed that I needed to make up for years of lost time, and my failure in educating myself, and lack of self-confidence. I was trying to overcompensate. There was this perpetual feeling that my past disorganization and lack of productivity was literally creeping upon me.

My mindset was: *"Today is training day and tomorrow will be the day to present myself to the world.*

I will change the world and produce! But not yet, I'm not ready...This musical phrase isn't refined enough, this film is shit, I don't deserve pleasure or the right to socially interact because I haven't graduated yet. I need to lift my GPA..."

This justified the pot and the Adderall. I would ingest a pill and for two straight hours I could write an essay with ease, edit a film sequence, run nine miles, practice piano, plan for the upcoming week. As soon as the effects wore off, the sensation of fatigue and sadness began to permeate through my body. I would immediately take another pill. This would happen more frequently as the semester progressed.

I was buying more regularly. I believed that piano, schoolwork, and editing were near impossible to do, let alone enjoy, when sober. The funny part was, as the piano recital loomed closer and I binged, I wasn't necessarily improving at my pieces. On Adderall, I would rampage through my pieces; bang the keys and desperately play the same phrase over and over without patiently trying to figure out the dynamics, voicings, nuances in passages—it was sheer madness.

I wasn't analyzing the themes of the individual pieces; the phrases, the lines, harmonies and melodies. I was just banging notes in an endless state of paranoia, counting down the days to the moment where I would appear on stage for my first recital. The closer the deadline, the more my anxiety increased, and my impatience and sense of desperation grew.

Adderall was only adding to the stress. It was no longer a means of escapism or elation.

When I was sober I wouldn't even touch the piano. I believed I was worthless unless I was high on Adderall. I had lost my genuine love for music. I had become a machine who only cared about perfect notes, like some baboon hunched over a typewriter.

I never sought psychotherapy, nor did I admit my inner turmoil to a soul, not even myself. If I had Adderall in my pocket, I would anxiously wait for classes to finish, counting the remaining hours of the day and five pills to carry me through. I believed that I didn't need anything else in the world! Life was golden.

I think there is immense pressure an Adderall user feels when on the drug. I believed I could only fix my life when I was high. I would go into submission when I was sober.

A week prior to my piano recital I willed myself off the drug to assure that I would feel the same bodily sensation while performing. I was fearful that the state of elation would be dumbed down because of my frequent use. My body went into shock. I'd been abusing the drug for months. This was my first time off the drug. I had barely any energy. At first, practicing the piano was torturous because I no longer got the instant gratification. Every phrase was flawed. While sober, I learned the truth; I'd been cheating the learning process the whole time. I didn't comprehend any of the pieces.

47

I had just been running through them, rushing to perfection.

Hilarious.

This was my first real glimpse of hope. I realized that Adderall improves one's *attitude* and willingness to work hard, but it does not make the work better or the person more intelligent.

I was a nervous wreck the day of the performance. I got suited up and watched from backstage as family and friends entered the theater. The concert was to commence momentarily; hearing familiar voices and scuffling footsteps, I quietly retreated to the bathroom to take my Adderall. My beloved confidence booster.

I opened the door and entered the stage. The applause sounded. I felt my heart pounding and felt like gagging. On the outside, I appeared composed, confident, prepared—or so the audience assured me afterwards. I started playing…

I had rehearsed and played through the repertoire on the program countless times. Going through it live, I felt some moments of joy. It was all muscle memory. I produced unique music I had never anticipated. I was proud of myself for having the guts to do this!

Nevertheless, I had robbed myself of a wonderful experience.

All the Adderall practice, all the preparation, I never once felt blissful or genuinely satisfied on stage. I was on amphetamines and while my energy and adrenaline were intoxicating, I knew I was not myself. I was not expressing music from my heart. I had cloaked my fear, attempted to conceal my vulnerability, with this ego-enhancing drug.

Accepting the trials and tribulations of making, experimenting, and finding music is inherently difficult. It requires concentration and patience. One must accept that perfection is impossible. *Trying* to attain it, the effort of risking is what makes music beautiful, worthwhile, and a lifelong objective.

I realized hard work done artificially with this drug at the expense of exhausting my spirit would shorten my lifespan. There was no way I could have longevity. At this rate, I would simply crash and burn, without ever finding a true sense of fulfillment. When you're plunking notes repeatedly, fighting the piano, fighting the given difficulties that life presents us—fighting yourself—there is no harmony. There is only discord and repulsion.

When I finished the concert, everyone stood up and applauded. I was relieved and happy. But minutes later, I was sad and drained. I remember thinking, "Do they know I took Adderall for this? Am I here? Is this really me, or Adderall me? I can't keep living this way. I'm a liar…why are you applauding this?"

After receiving gracious compliments and leaving the auditorium to change and celebrate with my friends, I realized how drained and depleted I really was. I had no desire to do another recital ever again. I felt like a part of my soul had been taken from me. I was finally beginning to accept the situation for the first time. The only thing I could think about at the celebration dinner was taking another Adderall, practicing and refining all my technical mistakes, leaving everyone behind. The next day I bought more.

This dreadful cycle of knowing I had to quit while constantly convincing and legitimizing my usage continued for the next three months until the final day of the semester. I convinced myself I needed to graduate on a high note. I set out to "master" 45 minutes of piano repertoire, have it professionally recorded, and finish my film thesis.

To me, these projects would symbolize my leaving the University on a grand note; on principle, to have found a love of music and a knack for discipline and hard work. Enduring all-nighters, followed by days of exhaustion, I was trying to escape the lies I had been feeding myself.

I now understand why opioid addiction has become so rampant in the United States: it's easier to pop pills and numb your pain than it is to face reality. "You are only doing this for now to get this task done today. Tomorrow you will quit," you assure yourself. But tomorrow doesn't exist. Delusions of grandeur or believing a tough choice can be made in the future is simply more procrastination.

In the last week of the semester, I was required to present my Senior Project to the entire department. There must have been 35–40 people present in the room. I had done my usual all-nighter piano routine and I showed up to the presentation completely strung out. I was talking a mile a minute, sweating, my pupils dilated to the point that I must have looked like a psychopath. While speaking and even maintaining a good presentation, I felt no enjoyment or sense of fulfillment. I was only praying that I wouldn't collapse on the spot and have a heart attack. I felt paranoid. My heart was pounding so fast I had moments where my vision skewed, specks of black bounced in front of me, like movie flashbacks or spliced images. For the first time, I realized that constant overdosing can lead to death.

Later that day, I talked to a friend on the phone. I remember bawling in tears on the floor, alone, huddled in fetal position in a practice room. My stomach was heaving and my heart palpitating. He affectionately said, "Don't hurt Cedric. Take care of him. I love that guy."

I had been hating myself for a long time. I had been experimenting with how much I could physically and mentally handle, what it feels like to feed the ego's insatiable hunger. I had avoided being around others for fear of rejection; always needing to be better, competing against others instead of trying to connect and work with others.

After the piano recording was finished, and I had finished my thesis film and had completed all my college courses and final exams...the familiar feelings of relief and misery fell over me.

I called my dealer.

We met in his car in a random parking lot. The moment was God sent. Or, I *chose* to view it that way. He said, "Hey man, I am no longer being prescribed Adderall. I'm not going to take it anymore or sell it." I think he was trying to save me from myself. I went into internal panic. How was I going to function anymore? I was so used to Adderall; the come ups and come downs.

I'd been through every trial that the drug has to offer. He continued, "Yeah...I've been taking these since I was a kid and I no longer feel the effects. I won't be buying them anymore." **This was my opportunity to be free!** I realized I was *grateful*. Yes, I could continue to go and search for more dealers and track it down eventually...or I could stop right now. Right now. I breathed a sigh of relief. I felt a glimmer of hope. I got out of the car and we parted ways.

The signs of knowing when to quit a substance you believe is ruining your life are endless. It's whether you're honest with yourself enough to recognize when you're going down a dark path. Adderall was no longer bringing me happiness and was taking away my capacity to enjoy life sober. You could say I was dying. I got lucky by not having access. And luckily, I chose not to continue and search for access from then on. Life will only get harder. I think constant drug use just makes life feel like an endless chore; a to-do list, something to get through each day as fast as possible. Rushing to die. And for what?

Post-Adderall, I've learned that every day poses new questions and obstacles for us all to recognize and overcome. I had taken Adderall because I believed I was stupid. I had low self-esteem and a perfectionist mindset that had forced me into a small realm without much support or intimacy.

For the record, I don't believe that Adderall, when responsibly used as directed by your doctor, is a bad drug. The side effects might be different or milder for other people, especially if you're taking the recommended dose. For many, Adderall can help restore order to your life. There is no denying the hyper-focusing sensation enables a person to complete tasks, time manage, stop inner negative self-talk and outer distractions (daily obligations, surprises amongst coworkers/friends, accidents).

However, in my experience, it comes down to what *kind* of life you want. All the trials and tribulations associated with Life's ups and downs are far more compelling and real when you aren't in a constant state of drug-induced mania. Adderall made me feel like a sociopathic robot. I wasn't concerned about other human beings. I was too consumed with myself.

Regretfully, I look back on my college years and realize I didn't create any lasting friendships. I didn't allow myself to be vulnerable, to have genuine human exchanges—which can't be nurtured with amphetamines. Those elated states only last a certain amount of time and there's something fake about conversations especially when you're the one in an inebriated state and they are not. There is potential intimacy in any human exchange. But if you're high, you both probably will feel that something is missing.

After college, off all drugs and medications, I began private piano lessons with an accomplished Russian virtuoso, Nina Lelchuk. I learned quickly that all my furious hours of practicing on Adderall had *not* made me into a musician. I had no technique. I didn't know how to read music correctly. I had no discipline. She asked me, "Why are you so arrogant? Who do you think you are? There's no discipline, no phrasing, no music. You're just playing notes like a typewriter." This was not to discourage me. It was to empower me, to wake me up.

I found that my dependence on Adderall had made me view life like I did music at that time; something to do and practice compulsively, void of love, sensitivity, or inspiration. Yes, Adderall made me focus. But I lacked the patience and never learned the skills necessary to create a beautiful phrase, to practice with care, to concentrate on the nuances of a musical score.

On amphetamines, I could not be calm or sensitive. If Adderall desensitizes one from feeling and being able to connect sincerely with other people, then using it to treat ADHD risks creating an empty, apathetic and purely narcissistic existence. It took being sober for over a year and a half for me to realize how selfish and narcissistic I had been in college. While self-improvement and success are very important, they shouldn't replace developing emotional sensitivity and empathy.

Perseverance and a determined attitude are infinitely more powerful than any pill.

Saying "I don't know" or "I hope things pans out right" or "it's not my fault, they made me do it" are signs of self-pity and laziness. Recognizing a problem is one thing, basking in it is another. I accept that I am going to have to get used to feeling vulnerable, even sometimes like an idiot. It's better to be wrong than lying to myself about how confident I am when I take a certain substance. I see that life is turbulent enough as it is, better to face it directly.

PART 6   Options

Big Pharma & Psychotropic Drugs

The documentary *The Untold Story of Psychotropic Drugging: Making a Killing*[31] suggests that psychiatrists as "mainstream doctors" have

---

[31] Burwell and Stith, *Untold Story*.

made it easy to access to Vyvanse, Adderall, painkillers, antidepressants, and other medications. Used to treat many psychological disorders.

From personal experience, it's easy to describe a series of ADHD symptoms to a doctor and walk out of the office with a prescription. I described my symptoms and walked out of the office that same day with some Strattera (a mild form of Ritalin and Adderall) as a trial run to see if the doses worked. I was told to ingest one pill per day and test to see which dose, ranging from 20mg to 120mg, worked for me and improved my ADHD symptoms or not.

It seems to me that any person could memorize and regurgitate some of the following frequent symptoms from the DSM V for ADHD to be prescribed stimulant medication:

- Not giving close attention to detail, making mistakes

- Squirming, fidgeting or tapping hands and feet

- Difficulty sustaining attention in tasks or activities

- Leaving situations when remaining seated is expected

- Not listening when spoken to directly

- Running, climbing inappropriately (in adolescents or adults, may be limited to feeling restless)

- Not following instructions, failing to finish schoolwork or duties
- Unable to play or engage in quiet leisure activities
- Difficulty organizing tasks and activities
- Recurrently" on the go" acting as if 'driven by a motor'
- Avoiding or reluctant to engage in sustained mental effort
- Excessive talking
- Often losing things necessary for tasks or activities
- Blurting out answers before a question has been completed
- Difficulty waiting their turn
- Easily distracted by extraneous stimuli
- Forgetting daily activities and routines
- Interrupting, intruding on others

Dr. Holly Lucille, from the documentary *Making a Killing,* says, "...one disease after another is popularized for the public to worry about... It's the selling of sickness. It's giving public awareness to minor conditions with the goal to sell more medications. It's not caring for people." "It is the branding of a drug for the treatment of a disease that did not exist before the industry made the disease." (Jonathan Emord, Health Freedom attorney).

Many therapists in the documentary described the patient-psychiatrist-pharma process as "trial and error." They believe people are being treated as guinea pigs in a massive human experiment by the pharmaceutical industry. "Lots of money is at stake and many patients want prescriptions for immediate alleviation of symptoms. Psychiatric tests are highly subjective and 'rife with manipulation.'"

You might assume prolonged in-depth clinical studies were done to accurately validate the safety of these drugs. However, drug studies usually run for only six to eight weeks!

"Psychiatric drugs can't be sold without a prescription, so pharmaceutical companies work with psychiatrists to promote psychiatric drugs to their fellow prescribers."

We are almost programmed daily to consider taking medications, either through word of mouth, by friends and our psychiatrists/doctors, or through the Internet and television. Lists of symptoms are shown and described through advertisements and this gives the person seeking help or relief to inquire about the drug to their doctor/psychiatrist. Just describe these symptoms to your primary care giver and you will probably walk out of the office with a prescription for stimulant medication.

Instead of getting to the root of disorganization and recommending non-drug

alternatives, it is likely that an ADD/ADHD patient will be given a drug.

Psychiatric Patient Advocacy Groups also promote psychotropic drugs: "You can take a survey, maybe sixteen questions, and if you're a normal human being who has lived through ranges of emotions and normal life experience...you can diagnose yourself as bipolar. So, you then take this information to your doctor." So, all you need is to correctly answer a survey to potentially get prescribed medication quickly.

The documentary then discusses "polypharmacy"; where multiple drugs are prescribed to counter the effects of other drugs. A vicious cycle of multiple prescriptions that can last a lifetime: one drug after another induces newer symptoms, to which there is another drug, another symptom, another drug, and so on.

In conclusion, in the USA, it is standard care that every patient has the right to be told their diagnosis, treatment options, including risks and benefits, other treatment alternatives, as well as the risks and benefits of no treatment at all. Therefore, it is highly recommended that you become educated on substances and demand to sign an Informed Consent option to be told exactly what your diagnosis is and what it's based on...and then what the treatment options are.

Non-Pharmacological Options

I suggest that anyone who wants to avoid or stop taking stimulant medications to seek professional advice from doctors and therapists regarding pharmaceutical drugs. Consulting professionals and familiarizing oneself about other drug-free options is important. Read books, articles, and watch videos about the effects of stimulants. Interview people who you know who have used stimulants.

At the end of the day, when you are sobering up and the stimulant medication's effects are wearing off, ask yourself, "how do I feel right now? Do I feel a sense of accomplishment? Am I feeling physically drained and shaky, rapid heartbeat? Do I feel a compulsion to take another pill in the morning, to repeat what I did today? To make sure I am productive again! Thank God I have another pill for tomorrow!" or "oh no, I need to refill my prescription as soon as possible or I'll never get anything done!" I think it's easy to know if you are developing a psychological dependence for it or not.

The big word here is *choice.*

This section is not meant to be comprehensive. I am not an expert on treatments available. But I will share some drug-free alternatives I tried:

- Teacher education services (IDEA, 504)
- Consulting with teachers and colleagues, asking more questions, taking the time to acquire more information and research
- Regular physical exercise (coping mechanism)
- Healthy relationships
- Avoiding abusive, stagnating or unproductive relationships
- Parent/client groups—CHADD, ADDA, and Independents.
- Experimental Psychosocial Treatments such as EEG Biofeedback, Time Management and Organization Training for School—Abikoff, NYU Medical School, After School Supplemental Training for Teens (Smith, University of South Carolina), Group Cognitive Behavioral Training of Adults with ADHD—Safren, Harvard Medical School, Ramsay and Rothstein, University of Pennsylvania, and many more alternatives.

I suspect there are numerous other alternatives to medications.

Support from Community: School

While I did not believe it at the time, I now understand that overall, I did have a lucky and supportive environment growing up, even though my home life was dysfunctional and high stress. Nevertheless, thanks to my parents' commitment to my development and attending a private school, where the teachers worked patiently with me, I discovered that I could be highly productive if I was allowed to be creative; envisioning and doing projects I loved.

I tended to succeed more in projects that required a storyline or a creative twist with the given prompts and educational content. For example, I remember a friend and I presenting a gangster rap song based on information we accumulated for our History class or creating a storyline for a family's budget that they would use on their trip to Hawaii, for Math class.

I think when a teacher tries to accommodate by helping the student complete homework and succeed at projects in an out-of-the-box way—it can help the student better understand the material. It can be through a PowerPoint presentation, a game including the material, a video presentation, a re-enactment through a play or script using the material—this does not excuse from tests and regular homework assignments.

But these can be alternatives and other opportunities to boost a student's grade and most importantly, to help them comprehend subjects without disparagement and public humiliation.
My self-challenging senior-year "WISE Project" at RCDS (writing, producing, directing and filming a story) shocked me into learning that I could speak in public, organize, work arduously on one project over many months. It was important to know for myself that I was not "stupid" and I had the capacity to create things and meet deadlines.

The first step to helping the ADD/ADHD person, especially children, usually starts with emotional commitment and dedicated support (in contrast to deceit, disdain and abandonment) from family, friends, teachers, mentors, and so on through a repetitive, methodical process. Rome wasn't built in a day, neither is attention.

Attempting to teach new skills at the time of an ADHD person's fear or moment of self-doubt can be counter-productive. Teaching new skills might force them to feel overloaded. Therefore, it is vital to coach them help them foresee tasks or projects to completion, but *little by little*, until they understand how or what to do to arrive at their objective and learn to trust that they can. If one section of a project is done correctly and they understand how to do that first section correctly, the parts become a whole, and the student can learn how to do an entire project correctly, one step at a time.

They have to be shown in the moment what needs to be corrected—but in a step by step process. Not an onslaught of information spewed out in a minute or less. Thus, if the person realizes what is wrong with one part of a project, they can assimilate and apply what they've just learned, and correct the rest.

Without developing self-belief, will power, and discipline, ADHD people cannot learn to foresee the future. The present is the only moment to improve. Treatments and forms of teaching must take place at-the-point-of-performance to develop the foundation of self-belief and personal discipline in areas they care about.

I don't believe in catering to a student's every whim because I strongly disagree with the approach that people with an attention deficit should be treated as "special." This can be very harmful to one's esteem, character, and work ethic, especially later in life. Ideally, parents and teachers should sit down with the child privately and discuss effective reward systems and explanations as to **why** it's important for the child to care and give effort.

When I was growing up, my teachers privately gave me pep talks with checklists for completed tasks, homework assignments, nondisruptive cooperation during class, asking appropriate questions that benefited class discussions, etc.

While this method can work, I believe *it needs to be kept private* between the student and the teacher. In my case, I certainly acted out and didn't always succeed at these checklist methods. I look back and I wish some of my teachers had pulled me and my parents aside, maybe had involved a therapist or counselor, and had asked questions at a personal, emotional level: "are there personal things going on at home? Can you describe your work schedule, when the kids come home from school? When do you all eat dinner? When does Cedric do his homework? Are there other distractions going on when Cedric is supposed to be doing homework? (Television, computer games, playing with friends) What extra-curricular activities and school subjects really excite you?"

Parents have a great responsibility to raise their kids; and I also think it's essential to try and get to know what your child is thinking and feeling, especially in those developmental years of childhood to adolescence. Sure, give kids structure, classes, extra-curricular activities, summer internships and jobs—but also, try and understand what the child is going through, what excites them, what bothers them, what family issues may be interfering with their happiness.

I was outrageously insecure and melancholic, so I looked for opportunities to entertain my classmates. When I received a check on my checklist, I would crack a joke about it publicly to the rest of the class. I remember in 5th Grade, the entire class had a pizza party because I had managed to behave well in class for a whole week and got all checks on my "good behavior checklist"—which I truly considered deep inside as ridiculous! This dampened my self-esteem terribly and didn't help me gain respect among classmates either.

When checklists are made public to the classroom, if your friends and classmates know you have "special needs" or that you are being treated differently by the teacher, they will most likely make fun of you. Especially in middle school. I therefore tried even more to disguise my feelings by acting clownish and off-the-wall, and I lost respect of many schoolmates as we all grew up and went to college.

I believe that if the child is taught that there are *reasons why* to improve and succeed, not just "because you're supposed to" then disruptive behavior will happen less frequently, or completely stop.

Personally, it would have been great to have my teachers or advisors to have had long term goal discussions with me saying things such as, "Cedric, what are things you would love to do professionally when you grow up? *Why* are you always being a clown and loud and disruptive in class? Is something bothering you at home? *Why* are you so desperate for attention? Has someone hurt your feelings? Can you think of ways to express yourself that don't involve disrupting others in class, and other creative activities outside of school? Maybe, another field of study (music, history, drama club, sports, etc.)? Where do you want to travel when you grow up?"

A *conversation* is what is needed for the teacher-student relationship to work, not a reprimand.

Perhaps unorthodox and creative methods using code words or communication signs from the teacher to privately remind the student when he or her is interrupting or losing focus in the classroom. It could be a hand signal, a facial expression, or a quick nudge or whisper when everyone is working on a group activity)—all of this would avoid humiliation by drawing attention from other classmates to the student.

ADD/ADHD people are often very intelligent with IQs in normal range or above. Just because someone has an attention problem does not mean that they don't perceive, aren't talented or sensitive. In fact, the sensitivity and high-speed perception may be, at the very root—from information-overload.

Support from Family: Home Life and ADHD

I grew up in Westchester with two great parents who are educated entrepreneurs. So, this is no sob story. But I can objectively acknowledge how a bad home life can lead to a child's melancholia and attention problems.

A family is a unit. Bad relationships negatively impact the whole family.

My parents were not happily married. Although they stayed together for twenty years, living nearby but separately.   I witnessed frequent disagreements and alienation.

Both my parents had work obligations and my brother, and I had multiple babysitters throughout our childhood. We would usually see our parents at night and on weekends and were around babysitters for daytimes and evenings. When my parent returned from work, I have many memories of them fighting and yelling. My brother and I tended to shrink away and play games to get away. I wonder if that also had a major impact on my behavior and development in those important early stages of life.

I think it's essential for the parents to be honest with each about their relationship. Are parents frigidly co-habiting "for the children" really good for the children? Is separation the better option? Is moving somewhere else better for the child to grow and develop in a healthier environment? Parents or guardians ideally should consider whether their declining relationship is negatively impacting their child.

In addition, my mother confesses that she had a hard time telling me "no" when I was little, thus, discipline was not established when I was growing up. Interestingly enough, she wasn't able to admit to herself until many years after, that she and my father were also not meant to be in the same household.

I learned to get away with things; not cleaning up around the house, having bad table manners, impoliteness, etc. My brother and I were happy and having fun, this warmed my mother's heart. Thus, it was very hard on an emotional level, for her to discipline me when I deserved it.

Ideally, a child needs to perceive that there is a family or guardian or someone who is dedicated to give committed, methodical, positive reinforcement during infanthood and through adolescence. When the child makes a mistake or acts impulsively, there needs to be a caring *conversation*, a dialogue to bring the child to understand what happened, how to improve, why it was a problem, etc. Repeated positive reinforcement within varying circumstances and environments is also essential to build the ADD/ADHD child's trust in the parent/guardian and his/her own self-esteem. Deservedly earned praise reinforces a good work ethic and encourages staying on task. And of course, rewards and fun activities are also great boosters.

While discipline in homework and home chores is essential, avoidance of punishment and humiliation is key. Friendships, outdoor activities, sports, musical disciplines, martial arts, studying new languages, and other extracurricular activities can be extremely beneficial for developing and strengthening attention in young kids.

Some parents believe in helping a child explore many activities allowing them *individually* to discover for themselves what they love to do. They don't force the child or put the child in pressuring or risk-taking environments.

If there is a disregard for competition and the subject of the child's health and education are concerned, there are no laws. Parents can choose to exhibit their child's strengths and talents or can help foster them until the child becomes older. Some children exhibit strong musical, scholastic, or athletic abilities at a young age and some parents push them in one direction. Some parents allow a child to explore many educational and physical activities, allowing them to grow in a way that is authentic to their nature. I don't believe there is a right or wrong way of cultivating a child's interests or skillsets. Everyone is an individual. What might work for one family might not work for another.

Hopefully, this all happens without verbal or physical abuse. This path of supported caring, direction, and discipline helps prevent against the child developing anxiety, depression, and other detrimental comorbidities later.

Healthy Relationships

Healthy Relationships are essential.

As a child, I understandably garnered a reputation for being a scatter-brained clown because I did not self-reflect enough. I didn't consider or care that, my desire for attention, my incapacity to be serious or direct with people, was annoying, sometimes outright disrespectful. My insensitivity to how my words and actions might offend another person were the reasons I felt dejected, found group projects (including my Senior Wise Project) to be stressful, and didn't maintain many relationships thereafter.

I don't believe everything is meant to last, but I do believe it's smart to reflect on your life sometimes and ask, "Hmmm, did I treat that person well? What did I do right and what did I do that might have been obnoxious or unfair?"

Throughout high school and college, I lost opportunities to make friends.

But I strongly believe that if a person has impulse and attention issues and doesn't work at being presentable, has a lack of respect towards others, then rejection is bound to happen and is quite frankly, deserved. No one likes anyone who is disrespectful.

I learned a lot from some bad relationships where I was selfish, and/or they were selfish. Being possessive, overly-emotional, and judgmental are not elements of caring relationships. I was too suffocating in some. In others, I allowed them to control, micromanage, publicly humiliate, and verbally harass me.

Unhealthy relationships need to end. If two people don't get along and can't work out an agreement or make amends by addressing directly problems from both sides, then the relationship is not healthy. Go your separate ways.

Psychotherapy

Psychotherapy helps extract and expose the mental fury and verbal dialogue from inside anyone who willingly reveals themselves to an objective listener, in this case, a therapist. This process can be very beneficial for the ADD/ADHD person. Verbal engagement helps bring awareness of traumatic experiences or self-imposed, usually hyperbolic, internal tyrant-thoughts.

We all store many memories and moments of nostalgia. Based on our past experiences, we develop ideas and beliefs on who we are in relation to ourselves, our environment, and other people around us. We may have developed skilled ways of defending our behavior in the outside world, justifying our actions and thoughts even if they repeatedly make us unhappy, near-insane, neurotic, and increase our feelings of being misunderstood and unappreciated.

Psychotherapy helps one face inner and outer challenges, differences, and discover compelling goals and tangible opportunities. The therapist-patient process enables self-reflection and personal growth through uncovering repressed anguish and discovering self-acceptance with freedom from negative thinking and tumultuous cycles of emotional turmoil.

Self Motivation and Discipline as Therapy

Motivation is key to success and overcoming obstacles. Nothing in human existence was ever won or created without motivation. I think that children with attention problems while growing up aren't taught to be concerned about long-term goals. They haven't had someone effectively communicate to them, "What do you want to study and do in the world as an adult? What do you want to try and offer the world? What kind of people do you want to be around, to be associated with, who do you want to work with? What careers or activities excite you every day?"

Without direction in life, there are no long-term goals, so motivation doesn't exist. It's not that they don't care about the future, it's that the foundation to visualize and actualize such ideas is not there. If you can't see it, how can you pursue it?

Over time, the ADD/ADHD person can become convinced that they can't handle responsibility. Others intervene and literally plan the young person's life for them because they have demonstrated that they are incapable of providing and planning for themselves. Understandably, this can leave an ADD/ADHD individual feeling very pathetic and inadequate.

In academia, attending classes, completing assignments, taking tests, participating in discussions is required to receive praise and good grades by their teachers, and eventually receive a certificate or diploma. However, the ADD/ADHD child can miss out learning from these life experiences and fail to see any point to these disciplines. I know I missed out on some of these principles growing up.

Culturally coerced and institutionally supported learning (pre-school, middle school, high school, college universities) place children in spaces where they are forced to participate, like it or not, with moderate rewards (letter grades, diplomas, degrees) and severe punishments (resulting in failing or expulsion).[32]

Over time, these methods of discipline can cause people—especially the attention-deficit types—to experience them as harsh threats of

---

[32] Larsen, *The Neurofeedback Solution*, 147.

punishment, humiliation, and rejection. This tends to harm their self-esteem and shape their overall character. They learn to expect and accept verbal abuse, disapproval, or even disdain. In contrast, positive reinforcement produces better performance. Tough love and demanding excellence is important, but it needs to be inspiring, not just insulting.

Thus, an ADD/ADHD child is more likely to be damaged by typical scholastic education systems and emerges perceiving learning fear-triggering and overly demanding, cause avoidance and procrastination. Learning becomes tedious and stagnant. Distractibility takes over.

I believe that when one commits to *learning a discipline they are truly interested in* the rewards can be great. This initiation must be in a subject he/she finds fascinating, requires practicing and dedication, which can help develop attention, "whether it be practicing an instrument, language, dance, sports, different subjects, poetry, novel, or work of art for many hours every day, and can spree confidence, newfound interests, perspective, and sense of fulfillment."[33]

Thus, I believe it's imperative that an ADD/ADHD person become immersed in many different activities until a few subjects truly catch his/her interest. Many people might think they don't have something they are passionate about, even though they did well in school because they

---

[33] Larsen, *The Neurofeedback Solution*, 147–148.

were supposed to. My advice: start reading and researching something—anything—to see if something catches your interest. Start with books on your shelf, or go to a library, check out news and current events on Google, videos on YouTube, traveling to some new places on a nice day after work, reconnect with old friends or family—Note anything that catches your interest.

Once a person falls in love with a study, an entire realm of exploration opens. Focusing stops being an unattainable obligation and becomes an enjoyable natural experience. When you operate from a love or passion, you become immersed in the learning process. ADHD people—heck—*all* people, just need to be *in love* with what they do, and order and organization will follow. There needs to be *meaning* and value.

Occupational Therapy and Primal Scream Therapy

Of course, I don't remember this, after I was diagnosed with PDD when I was two or three years old, my Physical Therapist noticed that I did not use my thumbs and had "sensory defensiveness" (I hated being touched by people or being in the shower). I had to be scrubbed daily. I loathed the experience, according to my parents.

Primal Scream Therapy with Dr. Elaine Haagen apparently was effective according to my mom as well as my pre-kindergarten teacher, Maryanne Marra. I vaguely remember my mom holding me tightly in her arms at these therapy sessions. I would eventually start kicking and screaming. She would say, "come on Ceddie...give me all your grouchies" which would only make me more aggravated. This exorcist-like process sometimes went on for up to an hour.

I would yell and yell and try to escape from the embraces and eventually, like a wind-up toy, I would tucker out from exhaustion in full-body sweat. I would go from a maniacal tantrum to a peaceful sleep. Doctors and my parents believe this was sort of post-traumatic stress disorder due to my being put in the ICU for the first few weeks as a newborn baby tortured with multiple daily needles for testing and intravenous catheters.

Neurofeedback

Neurofeedback is a recognized effective non-drug treatment for ADD/ADHD. A 2012 report by the American Academy of Pediatrics approved Neurofeedback as a level 1 or 'best support' treatment for children suffering with ADHD. Additionally, the Neuropsychiatric EEG-Based Assessment Aid (NEBA) System received FDA approval for diagnosing ADHD.

Neurofeedback, or EEG Biofeedback is a technology that links brain waves with a computer in a non-invasive way to balance thinking, feelings, and agitation. It uses sensitive instruments touching the scalp to detect dysfunctional or dysregulated brainwaves and helps rebalance them via self-regulation. It's as if your mind and the computer talk to each other. Your brain then smooths out and re-balances its dysfunctional or dysregulated brain wave patterns.[34] The result is clearer thinking, less stress, more concentration and attention—exactly what people with ADHD struggle with!

Despite positive evidence from (Neurofeedback) case studies, Russell A. Barkley, Ph.D., disputes claims that EEG neurofeedback has an effect on ADHD. Barkley told [*Psychiatric Times*] that EEG neurofeedback is not supported by evidence-based medicine. "One chief problem," he warned, "is that pre- and post-changes occur in subjects with ADHD regardless of whether or not they receive neurofeedback." Barkley attributed reported improvements in objective measures of ADHD symptoms (such as parent and teacher rating scales of disruptive behavior) to the practice effect. "Because of the lack of adequately designed studies, any effects associated with EEG neurofeedback may be due to the placebo response," Barkley said.

However, in 1995 a study by Lubar et al. provided comparative pre- and post-treatment measurements of several parameters in subjects with ADHD who improved and in those who did not. As noted, the pre-/post-changes observed in the neurofeedback-responsive treatment group were nearly equivalent to changes reported for pre-

---

[34] Larsen, *The Neurofeedback Solution*, 7.

/post-medication in subjects with ADHD. Other studies comparing the effects of EEG neurofeedback and psychostimulants reveal that neurofeedback produces post-treatment changes equal to those associated with pharmacotherapy (Nash, 2000). Based on these findings, supporters argue that neurofeedback achieves its therapeutic effects by acting on electrophysiological substrates of the brain and not via a placebo response." (Othmer et al., 1999).[35]

Dr. Stephen Larsen's *The Neurofeedback Solution (2012)* explores how it treats many debilitating psychological and neurological ailments ranging from ADHD to anxiety, depression, brain injuries, obsessive-compulsive disorder, autism, post-traumatic stress disorder, and more. According to Dr. Larsen, Neurofeedback can assist self-correction of brain function.[36] It helps harmonize the nervous system without using drugs.

Dr. Hans Berger named the brain wave frequencies detected with scalp electrodes during different states of arousal as follows:

1. Alpha waves (associated with a relaxed awakened state)
2. Higher frequency Beta waves (associated with effort and more focused thinking)

---

[35] Oubré, "EEG Neurofeedback."
[36] Larsen, *The Neurofeedback Solution*, 324.

3. Delta waves, the slowest frequency (associated with deep sleep as well as injury or depression)
4. Theta waves (associated with a hypnotic state, mystical experiences, deep reverie, and creative insight)

While dysregulated Theta waves are commonly associated with attentional problems, positive Theta wave states appear to open to higher consciousness from the unconscious mind.[37] Stimulant drugs, on the other hand, may *inhibit* theta waves, thus inhibiting this means to human experience. That might explain why I, personally, felt robbed of expressing myself musically at my recital when on Adderall.

Thus, it seems to me that Theta waves would be immensely important for artists and musicians, especially since artistic performances are associated with emotional sensitivity, creativity, and reverie.

In 2009, research by John Gruzelier, Professor of Psychology at Goldsmith's College, University of London, showed Neurofeedback improved musicians' performance. The control group did not receive neurofeedback, while the other students had neurofeedback prior to their performances. The judges did not know anything about the students and only evaluated their performance. Those who received neurofeedback training to strengthen their beta waves (effort and

---

[37] Larsen, *The Neurofeedback Solution*, 8.

thinking) performed significantly better than the control group, especially for sight reading and musical accuracy tests. In other words, Neurofeedback sped up their brains, allowing them to reach peak performance and adapt to the demands and expectations of the judges![38]

My Experience with Neurofeedback

When I was three or four years old, basic neurofeedback sessions with Helena Kerekazi calmed me down. In fact, the improvement in my behavior was so obvious that my father, Anton Bluman, went on to become a Neurofeedback practitioner and continued to help me himself. In November of 2004 at age twelve, I started treatments with the LENS Neurofeedback (Low Energy Neurofeedback System) with Dr. Stephen Larsen.

At first, I was extremely sensitive and could only tolerate minimum protocols. I would begin to fall asleep or get headaches within minutes of treating only one to two sites. My nervous system could only tolerate a small amount.

Dr. Larsen's mappings of my brain explained my pre-adolescent and adolescent states of mind from 2004–2009. My EEG recordings showed moment-to-moment jolts across my brain wave frequency band widths; indicating that my

---

[38] Ibid., 13–14.

brain was dysregulated across the whole spectrum. He indicated that the goal is to have smooth, continuous brain waves with less jolts and interruptions.

My brain waves were also irregular, compressed, and under-aroused. He explained that my nervous system's dysregulation resulted in disorganization, unpredictability (in relation to behavior and decision making), fatigue, and feeling 'scatter-brained.' These recordings corresponded to my attention problems, impulsivity, trouble following directions, and difficulty with organization.

By 2005, all my ADHD symptoms improved.

But the changes were not permanent. While Neurofeedback with Dr. Larsen was obviously beneficial, I was not able to afford continuing treatment for a few years due to my family's financial challenges. I found myself slipping back into my personal prisons; poor self-image, anxiety, low self-confidence, and procrastinating on everything.

In my freshman year at college in 2013, I resumed treatment with Dr. Larsen on a monthly, sometimes weekly basis. My brain waves positively transformed and with evidence of increased self-regulation. My EEG scans no longer showed spectral spikes. Sometimes a brief nap is necessary. Afterwards, I felt calmer and frankly, happier, more subdued and less manic.

Over time, I became energetically less sensitive, and able to tolerate more standard protocol neurofeedback treatments with four sites, whereas before I could only tolerate minimal or medium protocols with one to two sites. Following treatment, I no longer experienced drowsiness (common post-treatment side effect). My brain had become less reactive, more regulated, and more resilient. My brain wave amplitudes in slow to medium frequencies were also less volatile compared with past treatments.   I experienced restored impartial thinking, calmer moods, and improved concentration, focus and organization. I was told that my frontal lobe functioning improved.

This also corresponded to the time when I started to find a deep love for Classical Music.

In summary, over time my symptoms improved dramatically. I became less volatile and able to think clearer, plan and foresee goals on a day-to-day basis. My organization skills improved. I was able to foresee projects and plan steps to finish them. Positive thinking replaced my habitual negative thinking. I became less impulsive and felt capable of finding solutions on my own, amidst difficult situations. I do believe my improvements in cognition, self-awareness, and willpower are in part due to Neurofeedback. (However, I was unable to continue Neurofeedback for the rest of college. That's when my Adderall phase began.)

Problems with Audiovisual Technology & Games

It seems to me that external hypnotism, like excessive Social Media, YouTubing, Google Browsing and other audiovisual technology, results in the opposite effect from Neurofeedback. For me, it swallows my energy. Too much Internet and screen time consumes and exhausts my attention. It can be addicting; an endless source of entertainment and information.

I personally have to monitor and observe whether I am working versus when I am taking a break to check my phone; maybe I'll amuse myself with a short YouTube clip, or send an email. Because, I know, if my phone is near me and I am expecting a text message or a phone call, I will struggle immensely staying focused on an activity that requires my concentration. I'll probably check the phone a few times every ten or twenty minutes, anxiously waiting or checking for updates. This does not work for me at all and I can never get into a work flow. Thus, I have learned that I function better when I set an alarm for when I will next take a break, and *then* I check my phone.

Today, we are seduced into indulging in countless hours of flat-screen "reality" or "entertainment." Internet viewing has become another addiction. Audiovisual technology, such as smart phones, tablets, television, computers, videogames, etc. appears particularly harmful for ADD/ADHD people. I believe that by supplying continual distraction, watching "the world" on a screen for too long takes the ADD/ADHD person away from living his/her own life. I am convinced that if ADD/ADHD people were to stop—at least excessive—electronic usage, they would probably lead more spontaneous, enjoyable lives.

YouTube, as one example, is a goldmine of endless entertainment and distraction. Maybe you want to laugh and relax after a hard day's work:

Type in Louis CK into the Search bar. A variety of shows and excerpts of the comedian will appear. You click on one video and laugh heartily for a couple of seconds. Scroll down and you will see a range of YouTuber comments; people will comment on what quotes made them laugh the hardest, you scroll down and eventually a YouTuber commented something about violence, sex, or religion. You scroll up and look at the Recommended Videos beside the Louis CK video you are already watching. You notice a video mentioning Louis C.K.'s sexual misconduct and many other videos referring to other sexual harassment cases. You may try and avoid that, and you click on a Stephen Colbert bashing Donald Trump shtick. You tune into that.

You hear Colbert mention the White House's ties to Russia. You Google Russia and America on Google search, out of mere curiosity. Then you read a tabloid or search generated topic on Nixon and the Watergate Scandal, which reminds you of Dustin Hoffman and Robert Redford starring in the movie *All the President's Men* (1976). Then, that might remind you that you have a movie date with some friends coming up for that weekend. You scroll online to look up the critical reviews of your weekend movie, the date, time, and location, and then you notice Box Office Gross comparisons and keywords in Google Search, linking 'box office' and Harvey Weinstein, Kevin Spacey, and Louis C.K. Before you know it, you are now scrolling through a series of sexual assault cases and articles regarding Harvey Weinstein's criminal behavior. Then, you find articles of victims of sexual harassment, mentioning other A-list celebrities and their abusive behavior, reading various Tweets and Instagram posts. Now you've logged into Instagram and are scrolling down and down for twenty minutes, looking up trending topics from the day…

And in thirty minutes to an hour, you have gone from casually going on YouTube to unwind and enjoy a few laughs, to reading about sexual predators and the trending patterns of abuse of power and misogyny in Modern America, to Twitter and Instagram.

I'm not saying this is bad. But distraction and screen time are obviously linked—let alone addicting—and an endless source of information.

.;I think a lot of American culture and media teach the public that "You can have whatever you want, right now. You can buy this product, this phone app, this outfit, these jewels, go to this club, have this salary…right now" …. etc.

It's an 'if...then' relentless sociological programming that has made it so easy for Americans to race from one place to another, one person to another, one source of entertainment to the next. It's no wonder they call us "millennials" or the "ADHD generation."

It's a shame; walking through shopping malls, NYC streets and restaurants, so many people are on their phones. You can witness parents plugging their enfants into the IPAD or Gameboy — anything to keep the child preoccupied and quiet.

It's obvious to me: raising a kid with that kind of instant gratification and visual stimulation will decrease time spent perceiving and learning from living around people and the environment. It probably stunts the child's creativity and imagination. It also probably decreases their interest in their educational and social environments, runts interaction skills, and maybe even enhances antisocial behavior.

Let kids be kids! Let them be wild, interacting, questioning and have fun! But be there for them in the moment, modeling attentive organized behavior, incorporating disciplines, communication and education in their lives.

Of course, we want our kids to be attentive and not make too much noise, but please, not at the expense of decreasing creativity or dumbing down their spirit with videogames or innumerable iPad and television shows. Maybe they need more adult-modelling, caring, interactive attention to nurture and train their attention as early as possible in their development.

Spectator Life: Has Vanity Created an ADD/ADHD Society?

Henry Jenkins' essay "'Get a Life!': Fans, Poachers, Nomads," explores how Americans tend to dwell in spectatorship and voyeurism instead of actively living their own lives. Television and technology have seduced us into being spectators of sports, news, movies and shows we love, resulting in us living lethargic, depressive lifestyles of over-consumption and over-usage.

"The experience of watching television has become a rich and complex participatory culture where people are proud fans constructing their cultural and social identity through borrowing...mass culture images, articulating concerns which often go unvoiced."[39]

Leisure activities and entertainment are wonderful ways for people to communicate, relate to each other, and fuel social interactions. But such spectatorship can also be a source of escapism, endless time-consuming distraction. Now, constant forms of audiovisual stimulation are available everywhere we go! One by one, societal groups adapt, adjust, copy peers, friends, family, and even strangers alike in everyday life.

Everyone with a computer or mobile phone is solicited to have more and more apps for

---

[39] Jenkins, "Get a Life," 34.

shopping, music, gaming, email, banking, news, social media, etc., etc.—all our daily "essentials" and many forms of entertainment are instantly available. No one *must* think, read, memorize or ponder anymore. Quick answers are right there at your fingertips. God forbid you go a minute without your phone or computer.

As David Dubal, a Host of WQXR, pianist, teacher, author, lecturer at Julliard and Mannes School of Music, broadcaster, and painter, has infamously termed the modern-day man: "We are no longer Homo Sapiens, we have become the *Homo Mechanicus.*"

It seems to me that ADD/ADHD inattentiveness is becoming the current norm based on our new addiction to technological convenience, which will probably impede the intellectual and social development of our society in general. Isn't this the younger generations' mindset: "I don't want to be culturally irrelevant! I have to see, do, and experience what everyone else is doing and talking about! It's all about me; my story, my image, my network, my friends! My Selfie!"?

Our attention is being drained into focusing on body image and appearance; our proportions, angles, body fat, and so on. We are in an era where you don't need to become a celebrity to have paparazzi chase after you. You can take your own pictures and be the movie star of your own life and snap a million photos. You are your world, you are an amazing star in your own rite.

What you eat, who you're with, where you are, what you wear.

While exercise is very important for health (see below), it is all too easy to get lost in the pursuit of aesthetic competition while disregarding physical health and mental well-being. I believe that under-eating, over-exercising, and getting injured are linked and usually occur because of feeling insecure about one's physical appearance.

Being out of shape and feeling low energy and lame probably diminishes well-being, self-esteem and self-image, and may result in less job opportunities and lower wages. Not to mention, your appearance will usually affect how many "views" or "likes" you get on social media websites.

We are in a *looks*-oriented society now and our appearance, luckily not always, can dictate our lives and where we find ourselves working.

A major problem is comparing yourself inside your imagination to other people. Whether you think they are leagues better or more experienced than you are—or that you are vastly superior to them—it's all the same. Sure, it can be a source of inspiration, or discouragement, a compulsive habit, to feel inferior or superior to other people. Comparing and imitating means you never master yourself; you are comparing with your ideal image, and you aren't living your own life. You only feel more alive when you are like them, when you are thinking about them!

This is a major part of celebrity worship and a fascination with media. It's become natural to want to distract ourselves from things lacking in our personal lives by fawning after public figures. They inspire the public to reach for the stars and see that it's possible to be a worshipped human being. There are good and bad aspects to this.

When you are raised from childhood to "look up to" Michael Jordan, Roger Federer, Paul Newman, Beyoncé, Shakira, Hilary Clinton, etc. it can become habitual to spend many hours watching movies, television shows, sports shows, award celebrations, Netflix, videogames, telephone apps—before you know it, we are in front of a screen the majority of our lives—at work, at home, during leisure time.

This is why they call us the ADHD Generation. Everything is immensely fast-paced—just spend an hour in NYC. Our attention spans are becoming less and less, now we can only handle under minute long videos on Facebook before we get bored. A feature film had to be incredibly entertaining, constantly, to hold anyone's interest. Post a long email; it's highly likely the person will read the first sentence and skim to the end. This is all anxiety, rushing, competition.

I also believe concern over body image is potentially another very big cause of inattention. If you do or don't have ADHD, by thinking a lot about what other people think about you, you are taking time and energy away from tasks that need to be completed, or from tasks at hand that involve focus and effort. If we are concerned about our appearance or how "stupid," "silly," "amazing," "weird," "ugly," skinny," "fat" while performing an activity, then we can't be giving our best effort to what we are doing.

Benefits of Exercise in ADD/ADHD

Exercise is important for ADD/ADHD people because it improves mood and promotes mood stability. While I am no fitness guru and I am guilty of many exercise mistakes. For me, exercise yields a physiologically healthy "high" (I experienced "the pumped" feeling others have described when lifting weights, or the "runner's high" which usually occurs after 1.5–2 miles of jogging).

Even though ADHD children are hyperactive with bursts of excessive activity, exercise helps normalize and maintain their energy levels, slowing them down, leaving room for calmness and moderation. Exercise also boosts energy in the sluggish ADD person.

It also promotes better sleeping patterns and consistent sleep schedules. Regular physical activity naturally tires and relaxes the body. Regular sleeping patterns also helps an ADD/ADHD person to gain more control of his/her life.

A person can learn to pay attention and know what their body needs through routine exercise, whether it's yoga, calisthenics, gymnastics, rock-climbing, tennis, basketball, soccer, weight training, martial arts, stretching, dance, or other forms of structure and discipline.

Exercise can become an important part in our everyday lives. By improving well-being and healthy appearance, it can help self-esteem and self-image, which can indirectly result in higher wages, job opportunities, and promotion.

Yonathan Hormadaly, a "Rolfer" at Welcome to Gravity (Structural Integration developed by Ida Rolf) gave me some great advice: "What will help you, individually, function at your optimal level? It's natural to desire to do what everybody else is doing to feel connected. We all want attention. That's why we usually work hard, to receive attention. But you have to ask yourself *why* you are, for example, going to the gym and lifting weights (or doing other vigorous activities). Is it for health reasons, or aesthetics?"

Compulsively, I took working out to the extreme and then subconsciously distorted my reasons for pursuing it in the first place.

Take breaks! Stop any activity when it becomes monotonous or no longer enjoyable and switch to a different type of exercise.

Dietary Risks: Sugars, Dyes, Preservatives & Additives

What we eat affects our energy and ability to focus and function. I am not going to regurgitate a bunch of health facts and clinical studies proving the advantages of a balanced diet. But I'll try to summarize a few useful facts to healthy eating that helps balance ADD/ADHD symptoms.

There are many fantastic articles online about which foods to consume to improve ADHD symptoms and which foods to avoid, to enhance cognition and control hyperactivity. *Why Sugar is Kryptonite for ADHD Brains* by ADDitude Editors, discusses nutritional deficiencies or an imbalanced dietary imbalance that can increase ADHD symptoms. Following an ADHD-balancing diet rich in protein and vitamins can help improve attention control symptoms, but numerous triggers should also be avoided: excessive sugar, artificial flavors, dyes, additives, taste enhancers, and common allergens.

High sugar foods and snacks worsen ADHD symptoms. These foods can induce hyperactivity and restlessness. Trick words or disguised terms for sugar to look out for are: high-fructose corn sweetener/syrup, dehydrated cane juice; dextrin; dextrose; maltodextrin; sucrose; molasses; and malt syrup.

Avoid colorful cereals, candies and colored snacks. Substitute 100% juice and soft drinks and fruit punches, with natural, organic fruit. Most soft drinks and juices are artificially flavored anyway.

Also look out for dyes and preservatives. Studies published in *The Lancet*'s Paediatrics Collection and *The Journal of Pediatrics* suggest that some children with ADHD are also adversely affected by food additives. Jane Hoppe and Rena Goldman's article "5 Food Items to Avoid With ADHD" warns of the following chemicals and recommends that everyone check for the following chemicals:

- FD&C Blue No.1 and No.2
- FD&C Yellow No.5 (tartrazine) and No.6
- FD&C Green No.3
- Orange B
- Citrus Red No.2
- FD&C No. 3 and No.40 (allura)

Dyes can also be in toothpastes, vitamins, fruit and sports drinks, energy drinks, jams and jellies, hard candy, cereals, barbecue sauce, canned fruit, fruit snacks, gelatin powders, cake mixes, etc. Artificial food coloring and flavors, as well as the preservatives make some kids *without* ADHD hyperactive! Sodium benzoate has been known to increase hyperactivity. You can find it in carbonated drinks, salad dressings, and condiments. Other chemicals to look out for are butylated hydroxy anisole (BHA), butylated hydroxytoluene (BHT), sodium nitrate, and tert-Butylhydroquinone (TBHQ). Take note of the above additives and try avoiding them as much as possible and see if ADHD symptoms improve.

Tana Amen's "9 Food Rules for ADHD Families: What to Eat, What to Avoid" (2013) provides an excellent overview of the basic nutrients necessary to function at a high level. Staying hydrated and consuming enough calories and carbohydrates (but not too many) helps promote better physical and mental functioning. Include quinoa, brown rice, organic spaghetti, nuts, cheese, fish, turkey, chicken, beans, avocados, fruits and vegetables, herbs and spices in cooking, the list goes on.

Amen also emphasizes avoiding processed, microwaved foods, MSG, sugar products and especially wheat and any other gluten-containing grains or food, dairy, soy, and corn. She also addresses where the food is coming from (i.e. contaminated with pesticides or growth hormones), whether meat products are grass fed or industrially raised (fed corn, soy, and pharmaceuticals, and restricted in movement). Offer anyone with mold and focusing problems treats free of dyes and low in sugar. Best is homemade cooking, using complex carbohydrates such as whole grains, but there are plenty of organic products available.

On Acting:

On Camera Acting

Many of us love theatre, cinema, beautiful celebrities, stories and scenarios that have been re-enacted or dramatized for us to vicariously experience emotions and situations. We put ourselves into the film and believe that we are those characters, hell, sometimes we could envision ourselves being that actor or actress, on set, delivering those lines, lights, cameras.

All eyes on you!

I always had a fascination with film acting; watching my heroes like Daniel Day-Lewis, Leonardo DiCaprio, Peter O'Toole—I even did some creative projects of my own in college and checked out film acting. I began auditioning here and there after I graduated, got headshots, learned monologues and submitted various scenes to casting directors. I didn't truly understand that getting booked and pursuing acting was a full-time career.

Nevertheless, it was a learning experience that helped me discover what I truly wanted to do.

I composed my resume; studied the film industry, honed filming and editing skills, attended some acting classes in NYC, learned a little about how to conduct myself on camera, and to perform in front of casting directors. I later realized that the common theme for myself was that I wanted to get out of my comfort zone, not necessarily embark on an acting career.

In the film industry, casting directors, script writers, acting teachers—are looking for unique qualities in an actor's personality; quirks, tone, delivery of a certain line, the meaning behind their eyes, the swagger or quirkiness in their physicality, the way they dress, the shape and contours of the face — acting is an art form, a presentation, a lifestyle.

While an actor reads lines, converses, smiles, groans, contorts his face, expresses himself/herself, the people watching, taking in the performance, are also simultaneously thinking: "Ah, where can I put him/her in another production?" So many thoughts and decisions are being made in the back of the minds of the director, the producer at the same time during one moment of interaction.

And, of course, this probably happens in all professions, in all interactions daily; thoughts on top of thoughts on top of thoughts.

On Learning Acting

So, I eventually found myself going to The Actor's Green Room in NYC for a five-week course with Canedy Knowles. Each actor was required to learn a few scenes and then perform the works on camera, in front of the other actors to see as well.

It was a small taste of what it was like being on a film set. You have a designated amount of time to deliver a story, perform it with a camera and lighting on you in a close-up, and a script reader parallel exchanging dialogue with you, Canedy as the director, watches and critiques your performances, and helps you, the actor, better understand and internalize the character and scene.

You have all the attention you could ever ask for!

In the first few weeks, we were taught many different ways to "soak in" the material. How to infuse a character's associations with our own life experiences. To notice how we, individually, associate with and react to certain lines, thoughts going on in our head when we were rehearsing alone, when we were in front of the camera in class—all of this was done to help us better connect mentally and emotionally with our character, and ourselves.

I learned that these acting lessons applied to functioning in life, learning and performing music, writing, completing assignments, talking with other people, how to better compose oneself in a room.

How attentive are we when we are talking to someone? What kind of thoughts run through our mind when we are performing a task? Is it a negative thought demeaning you or the person you are talking with? There are so many subconscious, below-the-surface elements happening while we are doing one activity, having another interaction with a person.

In acting, it's essential for the actor to discover what his/her character *wants*. What is the objective of the scene? Through memorization and direction, the actor realizes that giving as much *attention* to detail as possible will bring out a great performance, whether it's a physical movement, a facial expression, tone of the voice, and more.

Canedy communicated all of these facets of acting effortlessly by simply asking: "Who are you? I mean, *you*, personally? Because odds are, the character you will play in a script and on set, will not be too far off from who you actually are."

This is called "type" casting. Every actor's dream is to eventually be able to play many roles throughout their career that enable them to create and re-enact different personas. But so much of what you bring to a role is *yourself*.

Hence, the way you behave in a room, relating and gesturing with other human beings, will reflect what type of characters you can play or how casting directors will cast you in projects.

I learned how important it is to try and pay attention to my behavior, the way I dress for a specific occasion, the way I talk to other people, the way I talk about myself, the way I behave in front of the camera, lights.

And the beautiful irony is that you can never get a moment back. Life is always happening. Once that scene, that closeup, that monologue is delivered, it's gone forever. Whether an actor is satisfied or not, the performance remains. All the work and preparation (meditating on individual words and complete phrases, memorization, choreography tone, enunciation, researching subjects revolving around the story and the character, and more) that went into that two- to three-minute scene, is there to experience in that moment in time, and only then.

So much of acting is being as present as you possibly can in the room, communicating with the people in front of you, including thoughts invading your head ("does the camera make me look fat? maybe the audience will notice I have pimples on my forehead, oh damn, I delivered that line terribly! This other actor doesn't think I'm a good actor! That actress is freakin' gorgeous—oh my God—").

The goal is to not give power over to those thoughts distracting you from what you have to do, in that scene, there and now.

On Practicing Acting

So much of creating a story, creating an entertaining or intriguing moment in time, is a process which requires many hours of concentration. If you care about telling a story and delivering a performance, the process of internalizing information about a character and the other elements of a story, takes many hours, days, even weeks.

I'll admit, the first few classes, I struggled immensely with memorizing lines, being present in the moment, feeling pressure that I had to "get it right!!!"

Alone, I found it interesting to plan out and rehearse every possible outcome; I would smirk at this line, gesture with my right hand for that line, raise one eyebrow during a pause, etc., etc. But when doing it live, things did not pan out the way

I thought they would. Sometimes it was creative, sometimes I got in my own way and didn't bask in the performance, the in-the-moment rush.

On Auditioning

I felt excitement, dread, nerves—all the time when I was waiting to go in the audition room, waiting to meet and sell myself to people I'd never met before, talking with actors in the waiting room, reciting lines for hours at a time—seeing 25–50 other guys sometimes in one room, all competing for the same role. It was all very interesting seeing just how much some people love the craft of acting, the fame and money associated with booking jobs.

Through this process of auditioning and taking classes with Canedy, I started to apply these lessons on objectively noticing how I was feeling about myself and certain interactions. I confided in Canedy about my moments of doubt or annoyance in performances, of joy, feeling lost while immersed in performance.

I started to ask myself, "Do I blow the thoughts I am used to thinking—about people from my past, experiences I wish to forget, things I feel guilty about—out of proportion? Do I imagine they were worse than they really are? Do I have to keep holding on to them? Or, now that I am learning to notice negative thought patterns when they appear, and to decide to tell them to 'be quiet' so that I can focus on an activity—can I start to form new, healthy relationships? Create new opportunities?"

Well, yes.

Am I trying to copy Paul Newman or Miles Teller—or am I going to accept that I am *me*? It's great to emulate and look up to great people. But to imitate and compare is delusional and very self-defeating.

Am I pursuing things I care about? Am I authentically making my own choices and behaving in a way that make sense to me, personally? Am I trying to be like someone else? Am I trying to be someone I'm not?

It was then that I realized that I was bothered by how, at this time in my life, all the time required for acting was taking me away from my time with Music. I really did not want to spend hours preparing or devote weeks or months to be on set or be "on-call," waiting without notice, at all.

Classical Music's Positive Effects on My Life

What Music Means to Me

For me, Classical Music has become a fascinating study that has helped my learning about music and more importantly, has helped me train my attention and work ethic.

I have experienced many different emotions through work with music. It can be an incredible outlet for self-expression, self-reflection, meditating or pondering about subjects that don't pertain to music and might pertain to other subjects, and most of all, music can be excellent for training attention.

I also genuinely love the sound of the piano.

I have had practicing sessions where I completely tune out the outside world, even forget about myself. I experiment with sound production, research and learn new descriptions and details in the score; immersed in the score in front of me, trying to learn and improve new phrases.

I have had practicing sessions where I was hunched over, hopelessly neurotic and practicing note accuracy, not making any music whatsoever.

I've had practicing sessions where I was lost in thoughts unrelated to music, banging on the keyboard, making no progress whatsoever.

I find it bitterly hilarious how one occupation can create so many ups and downs.

I often feel immense pressure mixed with sadness that there is so much beautiful repertoire that I will never have enough time to learn. Of all the verbally inexpressible meaning that exists in music, only some of it will be shared with an audience or through recording.

Music can make one feel life is not colorless, meaningless, hopeless. Sometimes, after I have a good practicing session, I walk outside, and the world is rich and beautiful with many wonders—the neighborhood or whichever environment you are in: scenery, the countryside, the chaos of traffic and city life, the tranquility of a small town, interactions with other people—the five senses become enhanced.

It can take years for a pianist to practice a work and feel satisfied or willing to perform it in public.

When a desire to express yourself appears, the message can come through the piece of music you are playing. It becomes obvious that attention is everything. When you care about your message and the message of the composer, attention and effort are essential.

When care becomes a driving force in life, attention and excellence become the goals. The process of learning can be slow and frustrating but knowing that dedication and seeing a piece through to completion—that is where joy and a sense of purpose is found.

On Classical Music Teachers

Unlike school classroom teaching, with piano, your teacher is right next to you, watching your every move, your eyes, fingers, asking you what you did with your wrist, your little finger, your thoughts about a phrase or an approach to a dynamic, plus focusing on the piano's sound, the music's tempo, melodic line, every detailed marking by the composer, and more.

During the learning process between teacher and pupil, there must be an atmosphere where both can be receptive to one another allowing communication and dialogue. I can't speak for everyone: some students do very well just hearing the teacher's direction and then applying it immediately; some students need other approaches.

If the student isn't improving then there needs to be an adjustment; either a discussion about how the student is approaching the work, what is he/she thinking about when practicing, whether the workload is difficult to balance with other life responsibilities, does the student like the piece, etc. When a teacher yells and the student isn't improving, it's a clue that the student may not understand or comprehend...or isn't practicing well ...or experiences frustration, fear, and anxiety at that moment. Once the student understands what the teacher explained, improvement is possible.

The goal is to figure out exactly what is blocking the student from having a breakthrough. However, if there is persistent/recurrent frustration for both sides, then maybe the relationship doesn't work.

Luckily, thanks to many teachers, I gradually saw how I get lost in my thoughts *while* learning and gradually was initiated into focusing better for a shortened period of time, 20–50 minutes, as opposed to sitting at the piano for over an hour, gradually losing concentration and getting frustrated. I learned when to stop practicing when I got tired or started to lose concentration, and when to return to practicing after "clearing my head."

When my passion for piano started in College, I was just winging it; I would hear piano recordings and then imitate them, playing by ear, without actually reading notes or the other details of the score. I would go with my "interpretation" rather than what the composer actually wrote. I would sit at the piano and bask in the sonorities and reverie, essentially, playing my heart out, but not carefully studying the score.

I've had piano lessons with teachers who were kind and easy-going, praised and ignored my inattentive technical mistakes. During these lessons, they weren't too critical and sometimes didn't point out my mistakes, and I felt good. But I didn't learn very much.

Then, I've had some lessons where the teacher hurriedly pointed out technical and musical flaws, checked their watch compulsively, and as soon as the lesson time was over, they rushed me out of the room. Their displays of apathy or impatience were very obvious. While emotionally upsetting, these experiences compelled me to practice more and take the piano more seriously.

Later I was fortunate to become the student of excellence-demanding teachers who train concert pianists. I've had lessons where I didn't even get past the first phrase, let alone the first page of a piece. Sometimes we didn't talk about music at all. We talked about my character; my work habits and my personal life, my future aspirations. I

would play badly and would be sent home to completely start over.

In recent years, I have had many impactful exchanges with musicians and teachers who have changed my approach to learning. I have been lucky to have incredible and intense lessons with accomplished concert pianists and faculty teachers from Juilliard, Yale, and Mannes School of Music, including many who have performed at Carnegie Hall, with major Orchestras, and throughout the world.

Here are some of the words from these teachers that had a great impact on me:

Jerome Rose (Award-winning Concert pianist; Gold Medalist of Busoni Competition, Faculty of Mannes School of Music, Founder of the International Keyboard Festival)

> "Who are you trying to impress?"
> "You were arrogant—how could you possibly think you can play the piano on your own?"
> "Nobody does it alone!"
> "Who are you, Cedric? What do you want to do with your life?"
> "If you can't hear the music, if you don't comprehend the score and what's written, you can't play it."
> (After I had just boasted to him that I had practiced all morning and afternoon), he responded: "Ah, but what *kind* of practicing? Were you paying attention the whole time?"

"The goal of piano playing is to play in tempo and create beautiful lines…to sing."

Nina Lelchuk (Internationally Acclaimed Concert Pianist, Distinguished Professor of Piano, pedagogue for over Fifty Laureates of International Competitions)

"Music is art of sound. Sound is everything. It expresses thought, spirit, mood, idea, character, energy, will power, and much more. No matter how loud or fast you play, sound must be beautiful, singing, long-lasting. Practicing is an endless process of listening to yourself, 100% concentration, attention to every detail. You must have a very critical, keen ear in order to hear yourself fully. Videotape your practicing. Perform as if you were onstage. Listen to it a few days later, pretend it's someone else playing, not you. Then you will hear all mistakes and faults."

"It's always much easier to hear other people's mistakes than our own."

"No one can concentrate constantly, You need to take breaks. Relax a while. Then returning to the piano will be more productive."

"You have to figure out how to touch the keyboard to produce the quality of the sound you want. The goal is to get good articulation, dexterity, evenness, and a real legato, singing sound. Every time, your touch must be different."

"Avoid any pressure over your palms, fingers, and upper arm. Watch your thumb! It should *never* be rigid. It must always be free! Use all the weight of your arm and make sure all weight from the shoulder goes directly to the fingers."

"Hands aligned, parallel to the keys, elbows in, curved fingers, wrist on the level of your knuckles! Wrist must always be free, using little oval shaped motions while elbows make circles, constantly."

"Use the upper part of your body, from the waistline, so your sitting up straight with the belly button as the center. Arms will always be in front of you. Move the upper body left to right with arms following the body along the keyboard in constant motion, making circles, elbows and wrist in an oval motion. This gives you freedom in your body. Playing piano must be physically effortless."

"Going too fast and rushing the learning process leads to no results."

"Be honest with yourself, self-critical—hold yourself to the standard of the music, the composer's intention! It's not about you, it's about the music!"

"Don't just play notes,. When there is no line, no nuance, no variety—you're just a typewriter. Nobody wants to listen to that!"

"To get a different sound, experiment with a variety of finger positions, ranging from flat to vertical. With your ear, decide what you like best. It's not just mindless repetition. It's an *artistic* process."

"Know music history and musical terminology
          —if you don't know a term, look it up."

"Desire to change will induce change: if you're stubborn and don't want to, you won't."

"Think before you play, before you speak—

think before you do anything—practicing is not about the number of hours at the piano, try to achieve more results in a shorter period of time, it's about productivity and ability!"

"Think *only* about music when you're practicing—about what you are doing—if you're thinking about something else, nothing will happen."

"Every finger has to work, with a clear goal in your mind. Ask yourself, what your goal is—the quality of your sound, phrasing, timing, evenness, smoothness of a phrase? Try it slower and lighter, crescendo, decrescendo…and repeat it as many times as necessary to make it happen. Intention is essential, then there is attention. Music won't happen by itself."

"75% of your practicing should be focused on sound production. Sound has a spirit, a soul. It has color, it can be bright or dull. Sound has taste, it can be sweet and bitter. Sound has temperature; it can be warm and cold. Sound has character; it can be very authoritative or obedient."

"Playing piano is an illusion. Good performers should bring an audience into a fantasy world."

"People come to concerts to forget about the difficulties of everyday life. They want to be taken away to another planet for a couple hours. They want to be in a dream world, a fantasy. That's why imagination is so important when performing."

"Don't say, 'I don't know!' If you have a question, ask, and find the answer."

"Your life is in your hands. You choose what to do with it."

"You're talented. Work with full attention; your brain, ears, and your heart."

Elise Cieslak (Pianist, composer, music therapist)
(While teaching me to sight read 4-hands music, she was the first person to realize that I wasn't reading the music at all. That I was only using the general lines on the page, but mostly following by ear, I was "winging it," doing what I felt sounded right based on recordings I had heard and not following the composer's notation.)

"Wait—what happened? You were doing fine! I can see and hear when you are thinking about something else other than the score in front of you!"

"It's *quality* of practice, not quantity."

"When you are in your own head, thinking negative thoughts or thinking about things unrelated to music, you make mistakes. When you are focused on the music you are just fine! "

"GET OUT OF YOUR HEAD!"

"Sensation of the hands touching the keyboard is more important than relying on your eyes when you touch the keyboard—when you perform, you don't have time to examine the keyboard!"

Ilya Yakushev (Award-winning Russian concert pianist)

"There was no particular event that made me feel like I was 'supposed to' go into music—it was a logical continuation of my studies...I liked practicing, I liked working on music, I loved music."

"I would not get so philosophical about that" (in response to being asked about the outside world while in the practice room, thinking about things unrelated to music).

"Focus on what you're doing at that very moment. Don't let yourself fly away somewhere in your mind. Once you do "fly away" you are done right there. If you feel you are not there (in the room) 100%, then stop practicing. Take a break. Come back to it later."

"Logic is your best friend!"

"Accidents that occur on stage or in the concert are usually caused by lack of attention when you were practicing."

"I belong to a group of pianists who believe that there is life outside of music—it's not necessary to learn all the repertoire...it's better to do less better than to do a lot badly."

"You have to find your ultimate dream...where you know that you are doing what you like to do and that you are happy in your life at the same time."

Rexa Han (Award-winning Chinese concert pianist)

"Don't let teachers tear you down emotionally."

"Study and associate with people who don't hurt you. Just keep practicing, you'll get better and better, you will see."

"In China, our main focus is discipline. You have to respect your teacher no matter what, it doesn't matter how good, bad, reasonable or unreasonable they are—you can never change the law—you always respect your teacher...you forget about yourself."

"Lang Lang is the God of piano in China: parents teach their kids, 'You can be a superstar like Lang Lang,' which is why piano, and discipline is now heavily reinforced in China."

"I can't represent everyone in China, but (as a child growing up) I never knew what I wanted, what I thought about what I should do...it was all planned for me."

"I have a strong personality and was able to make my own decisions, but many Chinese kids can be victims of the culture...I am sometimes jealous of American kids: they were allowed to have a childhood...I feel really sorry for many Chinese kids because I am sure they are being pushed into having piano careers."

"I like to travel, experience different things, I am intrigued by other people's cultures, food, how people talk—people in Russia, Spain, Italy, Amsterdam, Puerto Rico—the smell, the taste—and when you go back to your pieces, the Italian, Spanish, or Russian composer—you will have learned a magic touch. It has nothing to do with technique. But you infuse a beautiful taste into your work!"

"It's important to understand the world more...to live more."

Hyun Ju Jang (Award-winning Korean concert pianist)

"Sing the melody while playing the left-hand accompaniment."

"When chords change, try to express that something new is happening in the music."

"Start at the beginning of a phrase after you correct one or two mistakes. Don't just practice one small section too much, practice the whole phrase a few times and *move on.* You will come back to it later on."

"Notice changes and new ideas, special moments that indicate change, clues that you should change the Dynamics."

"Ask yourself: What does this phrase feel like? What is the physical sensation? Does it feel comfortable? How can you get from one key to the next? Notice what your fingers are doing."

Fred Boss (Choir-Master and Church Organist)

"Are you just sight reading (skimming through)?"

"Are you learning and internalizing the music on the page?"

"Know where the music is going overall inside each piece! Foresee harmonic changes."

"Imagine and hear different voices; a soprano, an alto, a bass, a cello, a violin, a clarinet…"

"Every note is a part of the overall color; every voice/note needs to be heard."

On Learning Music

Growing up, I was told I have an auditory processing delay. I now see that I misunderstood information being introduced because my own thoughts got in the way. When instructions were being given, I didn't perceive them accurately, uninterruptedly because I was being inundated by innumerable simultaneous perceptions, as well as potentially negative thoughts, all at the same time.

When I hear my own thoughts instead of another person giving instructions /advice, I don't hear their voice, I hear my own thoughts. When I hear my thoughts instead of the sonorities coming from the piano, I don't hear the music. Mental confusion blocks learning new things, new concepts, let alone internalizing music.

In addition, I now see that a lot of my auditory and visual blindness struggling with pieces was simply due to rushing. Rushing is the desire for instant gratification: not being patient enough with one's self, not carefully studying one's own response to the score, the character of the music, the movement and dexterity/direction or the phrases. Rushing also occurs when a negative internal thought appears.

If I am at the piano and I am rushing to learn a piece, these negative thoughts skew both my vision of my hands and their relation to the keyboard, as well as my listening to sound/tone qua][llity, let alone finding the nuances in the score.

Thoughts such as, "You're so stupid, how did you not recognize that chord progression or pattern sooner? Get the right notes, repeat, repeat, another mistake, you moron, get it right, get it right!!!" When you're thinking like this, it's very hard to learn anything, be productive, let alone enjoy the process.

My ego blocked learning and relating: I automatically shut down my capacity to take in new information, much like shutting people out in my personal life, for fear of getting rejected. I believe this is a major reason why people sometimes under-perform.

This maybe explains why new subjects that seemed impossible for me to learn in the past, maybe why I underachieved in school, why I failed to time manage—because I didn't ask myself five questions: *why* do I feel this way, *what* is stopping me from achieving the goal, *who* am I confiding in—a supportive or negative teacher/friend—*where* am I in relation to my goals, my passions, my living location.

So, my inability to sight-read music was really succumbing to feeling unconfident, and then blocking out new information.

For me, learning music helped me strengthen my appreciation of Time (time management of my daily life). There is only so much *time* to learn repertoire, practice, and then to share what you've learned with an audience (performing, recording) or your teacher.

While I have learned to think about the genre and style of the piece, the historical time period that the composer was living in, I also get inspired by listening to other pianists' recordings.

But I think it's essential to dissect the language and markings of the score yourself before you listen and imitate things another great pianist did in a recording. If you're trying to imitate others you will not learn the nuances of the score or the written notes and phrasing. That is your job to do on your own.

There are many things to explore and you learn something new every time you look at the score: Paying attention to the quality of sound, note accuracy, articulation of the keys, so that every note has a singing tone, evenness. Following the composer's nuances in the score and musical terms, pedal markings, slurs, dynamics, harmonic and melodic changes, rests, fermatas.

Vladimir Horowitz, one of the greatest pianists in history, said, "The piano is the easiest instrument to play in the beginning, and the hardest to master in the end." Sergei Rachmaninoff, also one of the great pianists and composers of the 20th Century said, "Music is enough for a lifetime, but a lifetime is not enough for music."

On Practicing Music

Through recreating a composer's work, a message is created for us to hear, an emotion or state for us to experience. Practicing becomes a genuine search—it becomes enjoyable and intriguing—like a scientist observing and searching for bacteria in a lab, or like a painter blending colors

117

on a canvas, a pianist is endlessly experimenting with sound, analyzing touch and the hands on the keyboard.

You start to fall in love with practicing, the process of learning. It becomes an addiction, a muse, something you look forward to doing every day. All the discipline required in learning music helps you realize that *any* activity should be done with care and thought behind it.

Planning which hours will be available for practice each day, then, utilizing those practice hours wisely, becomes vitally important. You can see for yourself when you're daydreaming at the piano versus when you're working. If you were daydreaming, when you put both hands together and try to play through a passage, you realize you did not retain anything you just "practiced." Wasted precious time! Hence, attention and caring about what you are doing at the present moment is essential.

Relentlessly pounding keys without thinking, without contemplating and pondering, digesting the meaning for one's self—that time "practicing" is also wasted.

I am guilty of neurotically practicing only for note accuracy or finger precision. I am also guilty of repeatedly making endless mistakes, ignoring them while practicing and not correcting them.

Over time, I have discovered two different types of practicing:

- Mental scramble, emotional hysteria, with self-destructive thoughts, doubts, and anxiety—all of which inhibit and ruin the learning process and performance.

- Patience, and hard work focusing, concentrating and memorizing—all of which create more confidence in playing, and better self-esteem.

Practicing has become interesting: studying where my attention goes, weeding out anxiety and impatience. My goal, every day I practice, is to distinguish what *kind* of thinking am I doing? Am I thinking about *how* to problem solve, or am I thinking about how difficult the problem is?

When you get tired, lost in your thoughts, frustrated, you have to get up, take a break and refocus, and try again. Sometimes you need to get the hell out of the practice room and be outside. Hang out with other people, do something else unrelated to music. For me, too much isolation is dangerous. Constantly trying to self-improve, I tend to become enslaved by the piano. I find it quite funny in a bitter sense; the harder you practice, the better you become—and the lonelier you become, too.

On Performing Music

Music is a mind, body, and heart experience. If the musician is missing one of these, the performance will usually be either technically accurate but devoid of meaning, inspiration, or musicality—or annoying, self-indulgent, self-impressed noise.

Performance requires weeks to months of time alone, practicing. Receiving the audience's applause at a recital, motivates and can help you to remain inspired to invest months of preparation and struggle for an hour-long performance.

There are moments of despair, too. Sometimes you believe your productivity is a measure of your worth as a person, so when you perform badly or with lacking attention, it hurts.

Interestingly, sometimes it doesn't matter what an audience's reaction is. Sometimes compliments, even when sincere, are not important. Your message and emotions expressed came from within you. Either you succeed at bringing that out or you feel unhappy that you weren't able to. That's when reactions, criticism, even praise, can mean nothing.

In summary, I believe that discipline and slow, analytical process of learning to read and play classical music under demanding but caring guidance can help people cognitively at any age.

Music training can "rewire your brain." It helps develop attention through listening, while being attentive to thoughts and feelings and their relationship to what's in front, what's taking place *now*, inside the room.

Even if you never become famous or make a career in music, your existence will matter to yourself. You will learn to care more about yourself, and can start to form healthier relationships, being more sensitive to yourself and to others.

When we care about what we do and what we say, we can bring beauty, harmony and meaning in our own lives and in return, contribute positively to the world.

Conclusion

ADD/ADHD is one of the most commonly diagnosed and probably misdiagnosed behavioral disorders. Many debate whether ADHD is a disorder at all. It may really be a marker for a different learning style, associated with intense perceptive sensitivity and creativity. For children, it may be over diagnosed since it is based on parents relying on professionals' diagnosing the child's behavior.

Of concern, the process of diagnosing it is subjective: one person might view distractibility as a sign of undisciplined behavior, while another might see it as a marker of a high-speed perceptive brain, being naturally distracted by impression over-load.

Another reason I'm not in favor of hastily labelling people with ADD/ADHD, is because it's incredibly easy to find some attention deficit, anxiety, OCD, or scattered thought process in almost everyone.

In today's society, it has become the norm to have (in no particular order) multiple careers, education, friendships, business relationships, financial and familial responsibilities, hobbies, social media, and other forms of marketing/networking. Perhaps based on our separation from nature and the environment with techno-information overload, it's hard, if not impossible to lead a balanced, "normal" lifestyle. We are all now *required* to have a multitude of skillsets, incessantly "multi-tasking" and "managing" Time.

If you have been diagnosed with ADD/ADHD and you feel the symptoms are ruining your life, it's important to confide in those you love and/or seek professional advice as to how to cope. Ask a lot of questions and explore *what* you want, *why* or *how* you feel scattered and unfulfilled.

We all need guidance in our development at any age, in any profession. While creative ideas can potentially be golden, it's important to have direction and to collaborate with other people to help these ideas manifest. Creativity and pursuing projects that one is passionate about is a "raison d'être" (reason to be alive) and I believe it's important to find what you really love to do and figure out how to pursue it effectively.

My Advice

Get to know yourself better and work at becoming your own friend.

- ***Find and Tame Your Fiend***

Self-analysis is essential (not self-criticism).
Explore your attention!   What is "draining" it away?

Discover, analyze and change your negative thought habits, become acquainted with the internalized fiend (thoughts of self-doubt) and recognize when IT is happening and ruling your thought process.

Your over-active mind is potentially a gift and *not* a handicap. Be more patient with yourself, seek guidance from people you believe can help you to tame and tell the internalized fiend to SHUT THE F*** UP!

How is your inattention or lack of organization sabotaging your performance every day?

Be your own detective: ask yourself questions all the time!

When I practice I'm constantly asking myself, "Okay, why is this passage unclear? Do I know the tempo? What is the dynamic marking? Is the passage uncomfortable for my hand, should I change the fingering? Do I have the right touch to bring out the sound that matches the style of the composer? What is the composer intending? What is new, beautiful, and different in this phrase in contrast to the other phrases that came before it? Should I listen to a recording of this passage and see what they're doing so as to better understand it? Can I play this passage well and am I ready to move on to the next one? Am I getting impatient?"

Be sensitive and kind to yourself: notice when your mind is wandering. Cramming and torturing yourself to do something you are not whole-heartedly into for hours at a time can be counterproductive as well as exhausting—and mean.

Why am I thinking about whether my laundry is finished? Why am I thinking about the car sirens outside? Am I getting distracted? Am I feeling weary? Maybe I should stop and take a break..."

- ### *Find What Genuinely Interests You*

I truly believe finding how much *passion* you have for what activities you pursue, prioritizing which projects to pursue and finish in a certain order, and your *attitude* towards completing those projects helps cure emotional trauma, raises self-esteem, and helps you find sense of purpose for your life.

Figure out what or who you love in this world, what you love to do daily, and confide in people who will, on a professional level, help you get to where you want to go. If you have too many things and too many "wants," prioritize them so they don't become overbearing and unattainable.

What genuinely interests and excites you? That you want to spend many hours learning or doing, trying every time to get better and better? Who rivets your attention and why (e.g. movie stars, philosophers, role models)?

Write down on paper, or record on your phone, whatever pops into your head constantly. It's a fountain of potential creativity! Don't let thoughts scatter you into humiliation, contained in your head! Whether you've been diagnosed or not—who cares? If you have a million ideas running around in your head, they need to be written down and potentially used for future projects, shared with other people. By writing ideas down on paper or recording ideas on your phone, they become tangible and they exist, not in your imagination. It also gives you a potential project to embark on.

Analyze your thoughts and behavior to discover areas of interest and seek mentorship, further your education, meet and get to know people who share your interests. You become who you hang out with. Be around people who make you happy, support you, who are smarter than you, who want to collaborate with you, who seek advice from you, too.

Healthy Relationships are Essential

Reflect on your life at times ask, "Hmmm, how could I have been better to that person? What did I do right and what did I do that might have been obnoxious or unfair?"

Ask yourself if/why you feel lonely, socially deprived, or have too many superficial relationships?

Is this relationship taking up too much of my attention? Is it abusive? Draining?

Do you have a good relationship with yourself? Take care of your health! The state of your body's health can affect your mind. Diet, exercise and avoidance of pollution and contaminated foods are important.

Be nice to you, too. Take breaks! Stop any activity when it becomes monotonous or no longer enjoyable and switch to a different type of activity.

▪ _Choose the Treatment Best for You_

The decision to take medication for a prolonged period is a personal _choice_. Pills can make a big difference, but they can become a vice of dependency. Not to mention the risk of adverse side effects.

There are many effective Non-Drug Options.

Pursue what you love, do what you love as much as you can every day. Strive for goals that excite you. Treat yourself and people well. It's an everyday learning process. We all have to work at accepting our quirks, loving ourselves and others every day.

Acknowledgements

I was extremely lucky to have engaged parents who consulted numerous doctors, therapists, communal support groups, teacher-parent disciplinary techniques—a plethora of attempts and empathetic research on their part for me.

I also want to thank my parents for helping me gather information on my childhood, and for their support of me in writing this book. I want to thank my uncle Jean Cieslak, developmental specialist who was the first to recognize my behavioral aberrancies and developmental delay and compelled my parents to promptly help me. I want to also thank Maryanne Marra, Doctor Elaine Haagen, the Blue Rock School (especially my storytelling kindergarten teacher Joan Miller who enthralled me with the love of creating stories, pictures, writing and drawing, and my first music teacher Joan Cornaccio who taught me to love singing and later piano), Lilian Boal who challenged me, Jan Flanzer, Ryan Berthod and Sasha Bluestone, Nadir Lameur, my RCDS teachers who worked with all my pranking (Mrs. Beers who cheerfully reigned me in as my first tutor and later 4th grade teacher, Mrs. Spira, Ms. Perez, Mr. Fyfe, Mrs. Eurell, Dennis and Marsha Predovic), my RCDS and college friends (Jake Miller, Nick Rocco, Osato Okundaye, Adam Kopec, Garrison Oliver Gross), pianist friends who were very supportive of my practicing and shared their genuine love and dedication for music (in no particular order: Junghoon Park, Tiffany Leard, Marina Simeonova, Julian Pflugmann, and Ziang Xu), SUNY Purchase College Faculty, Dr. Stephen Larsen for his encouraging support through my transitions, my other piano teachers through the years (in no particular order: Elise Cieslak, Rexa Han, Mellissa Alexander, Stephen Buck, Geoffrey Burleson, Quhyn Nguyen, Jerome Rose), David Dubal for his inspiring, story-telling eloquence, writing and mentoring, and Yonathan Hormadaly for his guiding my self-exploration , my editor Jeremy Lehrer, and Raymond Aaron.

Bibliography

- ADDitude Magazine. "Why Sugar is Kryptonite for ADHD Brains," *ADDitude Magazine*, Winter 2009. https://www.additudemag.com/adhd-diet-nutrition-sugar.
- Amen, Tana. "9 Food Rules for ADHD Families: What to Eat, What to Avoid." *ADDitude Magazine*, 2013. https://www.additudemag.com/best-foods-for-adhd-diet-nutrition.
- American Addiction Centers. "ADHD and Addiction." American Addiction Centers. https://americanaddictioncenters.org/adhd-and-addiction.
- American Psychiatric Association. *Diagnostic and Statistical Manual of Mental Disorders*. 5th ed. Arlington, VA: American Psychiatric Association, 2013.
- Barkley, Russell A. (1997). "Behavioral Inhibition, Sustained Attention, and Executive Functions: Constructing a Unifying Theory of ADHD." *Psychological Bulletin* 121, no. 3 (1997): 65–94.
- Barkley, Russell A. "Advances in the Understanding and Management of ADHD." Presentation, MIND Institute Distinguished Lecturer Series, University of California–Davis, Sacramento, CA, February 13, 2008.

- Beck, Melinda. "Mind Games: Attention-Deficit Disorder Isn't Just for Kids. Why Adults Are Now Being Diagnosed, Too." *The Wall Street Journal*, April 6, 2010, sec. D.
- Breggin, Peter R. *Talking Back to Ritalin: What Doctors Aren't Telling You About Stimulants for Children*. Monroe, ME: Common Courage, 1998.
- Burwell, Toby, and Randall Stith. *The Untold Story of Psychotropic Drugging: Making a Killing*. Los Angeles: Citizens Commission on Human Rights International, 2008. https://www.youtube.com/watch?v=rk-ryvdWPgw.
- Carnegie, Dale. *How to Win Friends and Influence People*. *
- Gaby, Alan. "Attention deficit-hyperactivity disorder (ADHD)," Chap. 281 in *Nutritional Medicine* Concord, NH: Alan Gaby, 2011.
- Gregoire, Carolyn. "Worldwide ADHD Rates Are Higher Than Ever, And It Might Be America's Fault." *Huffington Post*, November 24, 2014. https://www.huffingtonpost.com/2014/11/24/the-global-explosion-of-a_n_6186776.html.
- Harrison-Hansley, Milla, and Alicky Sussman. *Living With ADHD*. London: BBC Video Ltd., 2005.

https://www.youtube.com/watch?v=5lrcxmOol
B8.

- Hersher, Rebecca. "Do You Zone Out?
  Procrastinate? Might Be Adult ADHD." NPR,
  April 5, 2017.
  http://www.npr.org/sections/health-
  shots/2017/04/05/522711509/do-you-zone-out-
  procrastinate-might-be-adult-adhd.

- Hoppe, Jane, and Rena Goldman."5 Food
  Items to Avoid With ADHD," Healthline,
  October 13, 2017.
  https://www.healthline.com/health/adhd/foods
  -to-avoid#overview1.

- Jenkins, Henry. "Get a Life!': Fans, Poachers,
  Nomads" Chap. 1 in *Textual Poachers: Television
  Fans and Participatory Culture*. New York:
  Routledge, 1992.

- Larsen, Stephen. *The Neurofeedback Solution:
  How to Treat Autism, ADHD, Anxiety, Brain
  Injury, Stroke, PTSD, and More*. Rochester, VT:
  Inner Traditions International, Limited, 2012.

- Levine, Bruce. "Why the Rise of Mental Illness?
  Pathologizing Normal, Adverse Drug Effects,
  and a Peculiar Rebellion." *Mad in America*, July
  31, 2013.
  /https://www.madinamerica.com/2013/07/why-
  the-dramatic-rise-of-mental-illness-diseasing-
  normal-behaviors-drug-adverse-effects-and-a-
  peculiar-rebellion.

- MPR News. "The Tricky Business of Diagnosing Adult ADHD," interview with Dr. Jon Hallberg, MPR News, June 6, 2017. https://www.mprnews.org/story/2017/06/06/hallberg-adult-adhd.
- Null, Gary, and Martin Feldman. "The Benefits of Going Beyond Conventional Therapies for ADHD." *Journal of Orthomolecular Medicine* 20, no. 2 (2005): 75–88.
- Oubré, Alondra. "EEG Neurofeedback for Treating Psychiatric Disorders." *Psychiatric Times*, February 1, 2002. http://www.psychiatrictimes.com/articles/eeg-neurofeedback-treating-psychiatric-disorders/page/0/2
- Pierce, LuAnn. "Is Adult ADHD a Disability?" *We Connect Now*, 2012. https://weconnectnow.wordpress.com/2012/02/20/is-adult-adhd-a-disability-by-luann-pierce.
- Porter, Elouise. "ADHD and Hyperfocus," *Healthline*, January 27, 2016. https://www.healthline.com/health/adhd/adhd-symptoms-hyperfocus#1.
- Rabiner, David. "Attention Research Update: April 2014." http://www.helpforadd.com/2014/april.htm.
- Robbins, Jim. "Paying Attention," Chap. 7 in *A Symphony in the Brain: The Evolution of the New*

Brain Wave Biofeedback. New York:
Grove/Atlantic, 2000.

- Salamon, Maureen. "ADHD May Be Tied to
Longer-Lasting Head Injury," *HealthDay*, June
25, 2013. https://consumer.healthday.com/kids-
health-information-23/attention-deficit-
disorder-adhd-news-50/adhd-may-be-tied-to-
longer-lasting-head-injury-study-says-
677671.html.

Index